EMT
DEFIBRILLATION

Executive Editor

Steven E. Reinberg, EMSI

Managing Editor

Judith H. Demarest

Graphics

Edward A. Casker
Designer

Ken Swain
Graphics

EMT DEFIBRILLATION

General Editors

Michael K. Copass, MD
Associate Professor, Department of Medicine, University of Washington School of Medicine; Director, Emergency Trauma Center, Harborview Medical Center; Deputy Director and Director of Training, Seattle Medic I, Seattle, Washington

Mickey S. Eisenberg, MD, PhD
Associate Professor, Department of Medicine, University of Washington School of Medicine; Director, Emergency Medicine Service, University Hospital; Medical Director, King County EMT Defibrillation Program, Seattle, Washington

Susan K. Damon, BS, RN
EMT Defibrillation Program Coordinator, King County Emergency Medical Services Division, King County Department of Health, Seattle, Washington

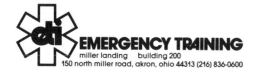

EMERGENCY TRAINING
miller landing   building 200
150 north miller road, akron, ohio 44313 (216) 836-0600

Acknowledgments

The efforts of many individuals contributed to this text. Ken Stults provided material for the section on EMT Defibrillation in rural communities. Barbara Blake, RN, and Robbi Galbraith assisted in curriculum development. Sue Edwards and the Medic I training office helped coordinate early training sessions. Judy Prentice and Harriet Moles graciously typed our numerous drafts of the manuscript. Invaluable assistance in all aspects of training was provided by Tom Torell. Numerous paramedics and fire chiefs have directly assisted in the training program.

Our highest respect and appreciation go to the several hundred EMTs of Seattle and King County who volunteered their time and who demonstrated that dedication and professionalism can make the impossible possible.

Development of the EMT Defibrillation program in King County, Washington was supported by a grant from The National Center for Health Services Research, grant number (HS 03215).

This book is dedicated to the thousands of Emergency Medical Technicians and Paramedics whose devotion to learning the skills of emergency care enable them to pluck life from the jaws of death.

Printed in the United States of America   ISBN 0-940432-04-8

Curriculum Guidelines

The cardiac rhythms that the EMT-D must master are:
Normal Sinus Rhythm
Ventricular Tachycardia
Ventricular Flutter
Ventricular Fibrillation
Asystole

The basic decision faced by the EMT-D is whether the rhythm is ventricular fibrillation or something else. If the rhythm is not ventricular fibrillation it is not mandatory that it be identified by name.

This text includes more material than is necessary for the EMT-D to master. The additional material consists of:
Sinus Bradycardia
Sinus Arrhythmia
Sinus Tachycardia
Atrial Flutter
Atrial Fibrillation
Nodal Rhythm
Heart Blocks
Premature Ventricular Contractions
Idioventricular Rhythm

This additional material is included for the more motivated student, and should be considered optional.

Contents

Preface

There is nothing more dramatic than sudden cardiac arrest. An individual, often in good health with no known serious illness, may, in a matter of seconds, suddenly collapse. There may be no warning symptoms. Symptoms, if present, may be present for only seconds. The person may experience dizziness or a sense of impending doom. The individual collapses; consciousness is lost, pulse ceases, blood pressure falls to zero. Agonal, gasping respirations may continue for 30 seconds to a minute; but these soon cease. As the brain is deprived of oxygen, there may be a seizure and incontinence of stool or urine. At the moment the pulse and blood pressure fall to zero the cells are deprived of oxygen, and acidosis begins. Organ and brain damage become irreversible in a short four minutes. If circulation is not maintained, this individual becomes irretrievably dead: another statistic tolling the large numbers of persons dying from cardiovascular disease.

As an Emergency Medical Technician, you've been trained to deal with and initiate therapy for many life-threatening conditions and emergency problems. However, for the most dramatic and urgent of medical emergencies — sudden cardiac arrest — there has been little an Emergency Medical Technician could do other than initiate and provide cardiopulmonary resuscitation. Cardiopulmonary resuscitation, while vital to maintaining circulation to the body, rarely converts a heart in cardiac arrest into a spontaneously beating heart. CPR buys time until more definitive care can be brought to the patient. The purpose of EMT defibrillation is to provide the EMT and the Intermediate EMT with a true lifesaving skill for patients who have sudden cardiac arrest.

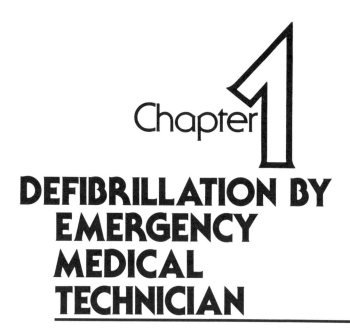

Chapter 1

DEFIBRILLATION BY EMERGENCY MEDICAL TECHNICIAN

This textbook has been written to provide you with the knowledge and skills necessary to operate a defibrillator and the ability to recognize cardiac rhythms so that you will know when the machine is to be used. Training in EMT defibrillation should not be undertaken lightly. While it offers a significant chance to save a life, it also has great potential to be harmful not only to a patient but to the EMT as well.

To set the stage and to emphasize the importance of the material contained in the text, we have listed the Ten Commandments of EMT defibrillation. The commandments must never be violated.

EMT Defibrillation Ten Commandments

1. Thou shalt save a life. Indeed, the entire purpose of this training is to provide the EMT with the capacity to save a life. To provide therapy for a person in cardiac arrest who is dead by using an electric shock to jolt the heart into a life-sustaining rhythm is one of the most gratifying experiences imaginable. If EMTs with defibrillators can arrive in time at the scene of a cardiac arrest, there is an excellent chance that lives will be saved.

2. Thou shalt act professionally. Encountering death is a humbling experience. Death is something we know we must all face ourselves. It is not to be treated with disrespect. An EMT at the scene of a cardiac arrest must be a professional and treat the situation with dignity and the relatives and bystanders with respect and compassion. Don't be afraid to show your sympathy to relatives. Realize that grief on their part is natural. Be supportive and helpful in every way you can.

Not everyone in cardiac arrest can be brought back to life even if EMT defibrillation arrives immediately. Some people will have severe underlying disease, or will have suffered previous myocardial infarctions, or will have a terminal disease such as cancer. Perhaps the interval will be too long for defibrillation to be of benefit. Whatever the reason, realize that only some lives will be saved; not all of them. The best estimate as to the number of lives likely to be saved is approximately one in five if EMT defibrillation skills can be brought to the scene within approximately 5–10 minutes from time of collapse.

3. Thou shalt never ignore the patient. Never forget your basic skills as an EMT. They include assessment of the patient's condition and determination of vital signs. Most of the cases you treat will not be in cardiac arrest; don't forget basic patient assessment. Even in cases of cardiac arrest, continued patient assessment is of paramount importance. Obtain vital signs frequently and keep your attention focused on the patient. Initiate CPR rapidly if vital signs are absent. Don't focus on the defibrillator machine. The defibrillator is only a tool to assist you *after* you have determined that cardiac arrest is present.

4. Thou shalt follow standing orders. Standing orders authorize you to use a defibrillator. They must be followed to the letter. The orders protect you from legal liability. If you act in accordance with the orders it is unlikely that you will be legally at risk. If you deviate from the orders you may find yourself vulnerable to litigation. The standing orders also protect the doctor. EMT defibrillation is considered an extension of the physician's medical practice license in most states. Hence, for you to be a legal extension of the physician's practice, you must be authorized in writing. This authorization is what we call "standing orders."

5. Thou shalt know ventricular fibrillation with all your heart. Ventricular fibrillation is the heart rhythm that can be successfully treated with defibrillation. This rhythm must be distinguished from all other rhythms. This training will provide you with the ability to recognize ventricular fibrillation and distinguish it from other heart rhythms.

6. Thou shalt act fast. The major benefit of defibrillation occurs when it is delivered to the patient quickly. The longer the interval from collapse to first shock, the less likely it is that the person will be saved. There is a strong relationship between response time and the likelihood of successful resuscitation. For every minute that can be shaved from response time another 5–10% of cardiac arrest patients can be saved. Once an EMT is at the scene, he/she must act rapidly in making the decision to utilize the defibrillator.

7. Thou shalt act cautiously. Although the sixth commandment is to act fast, you must also act cautiously. Reckless haste places the EMT and the patient in jeopardy. An unnecessary defibrillation can kill a patient. Careless use of the equipment can harm the EMT.

8. Thou shalt document the care you give. For an EMT Defibrillation Program to be operated safely, there must be medical supervision. Medical supervision requires accurate documentation of what was done, when it was done, and who did it. Complete and accurate run reports must be completed following EMT defibrillation treatment. We also strongly recommend that there be documented evidence of the patient's cardiac rhythm, pre- and post-defibrillation. Ideally, this can be obtained with an ECG rhythm strip as well as with a cassette tape recorder. Some cassette tape recorders are available that can record both the patient's heart rhythm and the voices of the EMTs at the scene. In such situations the EMT must speak up and give a verbal commentary throughout the resuscitation.

9. Thou shalt maintain the equipment. A defibrillator is as vital a piece of equipment as a $200,000 fire truck pumper or a $30,000 ambulance. It will not do one bit of good if it is not in perfect working order. To be in perfect working order it requires daily maintenance checks. The machines must be treated with care. Most defibrillators on the market cost approximately $7,000.

10. Thou shalt never screw up. Obvious, isn't it?

Cardiac Arrest: Who Shall Live? Who Shall Die?

Studies in the last decade have identified factors that determine whether an individual survives following cardiac arrest. Some of these are called *fate factors,* and some are *system factors.*

FATE FACTORS

These are factors that are not determined by the Emergency Medicine Service System, but rather have to do with chance or fate. For example, the age of the person is important in determining survival or death following cardiac arrest. Individuals in their 50s and early 60s are more likely to survive than individuals in their 70s or 80s.

Another important fate factor is the person's underlying medical condition. If the patient has severe underlying medical problems such as advanced heart failure or widespread cancer, then no therapy, no matter how timely, is likely to be of benefit.

A third important fate factor is whether the collapse of the person is witnessed directly. If a friend, relative, or bystander sees the person collapse, then, of course, emergency help is more likely to be administered in a short period of time. On the other hand, if a person is discovered already collapsed, perhaps for several minutes or longer, then the odds of successful resuscitation fall dramatically.

A fourth important fate factor is the cardiac rhythm that causes the cardiac arrest. If a person has ventricular fibrillation (which is the most common cause of cardiac arrest) there is high likelihood of successful resuscitation if defibrillation can be delivered rapidly. If the rhythm causing cardiac arrest is not ventricular fibrillation, there is a very small likelihood of successful resuscitation.

SYSTEM FACTORS

As important as fate factors are the *system factors.* System factors have to do with the kind of emergency care available in the community. These factors do much to determine whether an individual lives or dies. An important system factor is the time from collapse to CPR. If this interval is four minutes or less, the individual has a high likelihood of successful resuscitation. Clearly, if the community has many citizens trained in CPR, and if a citizen starts CPR prior to emergency agency arrival, then this time will be short and the patient will have a higher chance of resuscitation. If aid units or rescue vehicles can arrive at the scene rapidly to start CPR, then again, the patient will have a high likelihood of resuscitation.

The second important system factor is the time from collapse to definitive cardiac care. CPR buys time, but definitive care provides the actual treatment that converts a heart in arrest to one with a life-sustaining rhythm. The most important element of definitive cardiac care is defibrillation. If a defibrillatory shock can be provided to the heart rapidly enough this treatment alone may be sufficient to establish a life-sustaining rhythm. The patient may not immediately require medications to maintain the heart's rhythm. In many communities, definitive care with defibrillation is provided by paramedics. In communities without paramedics, Emergency Medical Technicians (assuming they could not defibrillate) must transport the patients to the hospital where definitive care is provided. The purpose of EMT defibrillation is to give EMTs this vital skill so that it can be brought to the patient rapidly and improve the chances of resuscitation.

If CPR can be started within four minutes and if definitive care *(defibrillation)* can be provided within 8–10 minutes, about two out of five patients will be successfully resuscitated and discharged alive from the hospital following sudden cardiac arrest.

History of EMT Defibrillation

A pilot program using EMT defibrillation was initiated in King County, Washington, in 1978. Until 1978, the Auburn–Federal Way community in King County had basic Emergency Medical Technician services. Patients in cardiac arrest had CPR initiated at the scene by a bystander or the emergency agency personnel and were then transported to the hospital, with ongoing CPR, for definitive care (such as defibrillation). Because of the time from collapse to provision of definitive care (average 21 minutes) very few cardiac arrest patients survived (less than 4%). Beginning in 1978, all emergency agencies in the area provided defibrillation by Emergency Medical Technicians. Eleven emergency vehicles were equipped with defibrillators. Fifty EMTs were trained and certified in the use of a defibrillator. During the one-year period when this new service was available, almost 20% of the cardiac arrest patients survived out-of-hospital cardiac arrest and were discharged alive from the hospital. A major reason accounting for this five-fold improvement was the fact that the time from collapse to provision of defibrillatory shocks fell from 21 minutes to six minutes when the EMT defibrillation services were available.

Because of the success with the pilot program, EMT defibrillation (EMT-D) services began in other parts of the country as well as the city of Seattle. Experience with these programs has shown repeatedly that EMT defibrillation is life-saving and that it improves the chances of survival when compared to basic EMT services. Based upon the positive experiences in Seattle and King County, the program has received state approval and many communities throughout Washington now have EMT defibrillation programs. Since then, other communities throughout the nation have initiated these programs, and interest in them on the part of EMTs and emergency agency directors has grown steadily.

EMT defibrillation services are not intended to replace paramedic services. Paramedics, in general, receive hundreds of hours of training and have the knowledge and skills to provide far more than defibrillatory shocks. Paramedics are trained to provide emergency medications, establish intravenous access, and perform esophageal or endotracheal intubation. Indeed, many patients in cardiac arrest cannot be saved with defibrillation alone, but require medications and other advanced procedures. EMT defibrillation services should never be viewed as a replacement for paramedic services. Where paramedic services exist, EMT defibrillation may supplement emergency care so that even higher resuscitation rates can occur.

COMMUNITIES LIKELY TO BENEFIT FROM EMT-D

From the King County and Seattle experiences, a picture has emerged that identifies communities likely to benefit from EMT defibrillation services. For communities with only basic EMT services, an EMT Defibrillation Program is likely to save lives if the average EMT response time is approximately 6–10 minutes. If this response time is greater than 10 minutes, an EMT Defibrillation Program is unlikely to save many lives. For communities that already have paramedic programs, EMT defibrillation can supplement and enhance paramedic programs, particularly if the interval between EMT and paramedic arrival is greater than 4 minutes. In other words, in communities with tiered response systems (with EMTs providing first care and paramedics arriving several minutes later) EMT defibrillation service can be of benefit since the initial shock is provided prior to the paramedics' arrival.

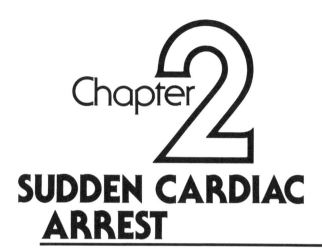

Chapter 2

SUDDEN CARDIAC ARREST

Heart disease is the greatest killer of adults in the United States. Over 650,000 persons die annually from heart disease in the United States. Approximately half (350,000) die before they even reach the hospital. The fact that so many individuals die suddenly in their homes and places of work has been the major reason for the development of Emergency Medical Services and EMT and Paramedic Programs. It was demonstrated in the early '70s that if advanced medical skills were taken directly to collapsed individuals, lives could be saved.

Causes of Sudden Cardiac Arrest

Because of the large numbers dying annually from heart disease, a great deal of scientific and medical attention has been devoted to defining the causes of cardiac arrest. While much is known, there is still much that needs to be understood. Sudden cardiac arrest usually occurs in individuals in their 50s and 60s although it may occur less commonly in individuals in their 30s to 40s. It is three times more common in men than in women. Persons who have sudden cardiac arrest usually have underlying arteriosclerotic heart disease (hardening of the arteries). Arteriosclerosis is a slow, progressive disease; it may begin in the teenage years and continue slowly into adulthood. In arteriosclerosis the walls of the arteries become thickened with deposits of fatty substances such as cholesterol. As the arteries become narrowed, the blood supply to various parts of the body is reduced. If the narrowing becomes too great or the vessel becomes blocked, then that portion of the body which is supplied by the artery is irreparably damaged. If the arteries of the heart are involved and if one of them becomes blocked, then that portion of the heart supplied by the artery is damaged. This is what is known as a myocardial infarction, or heart attack. Thus, in a heart attack a block occurs in one of the arteries directly supplying blood to the heart muscle. When the blood supply becomes blocked, that portion of the heart muscle begins to die. If the heart muscle is starved of oxygen and nutrients, then the muscle cannot function properly. Damaged muscle releases acids, which cause an area of irritability. This in turn causes the heart's normal pumping rhythm to become very abnormal. If the abnormal rhythm is ventricular fibrillation, then no blood is pumped out to the body. This is sudden cardiac arrest.

Another way in which sudden cardiac arrest may occur is through electrical death. In this situation a heart attack does not occur but, for reasons which are not well understood, the heart's normal rhythm suddenly turns into a fatal rhythm (in most instances, ventricular fibrillation). This sudden change from a normal rhythm to a fatal rhythm also results in sudden cardiac arrest. Although persons with sudden cardiac arrest have underlying arteriosclerosis, only one-third have an actual heart attack. The others have their arrest due to an electrical disturbance. The result, however, is the same. A heart that was normally pumping blood to the body suddenly stops because of the disturbance in rhythm, and unless definitive care is provided quickly, the person will die.

Candidates for Sudden Cardiac Arrest

Many factors contribute to the development of arteriosclerosis and heart attacks.
1. High blood pressure, if it is not controlled with medication, is a very strong contributing factor to the development of a heart attack.
2. Cigarette smoking has been shown to contribute to the development of arteriosclerosis and heart disease.
3. Very high levels of cholesterol contribute to the development of arteriosclerosis.
4. Individuals with diabetes are more likely to have early onset of arteriosclerosis.
5. Persons whose fathers or mothers died of heart disease are more likely themselves to develop arteriosclerosis than persons who did not have a family history of heart disease.
6. Lack of exercise, excess weight, and a stressful life style have been shown in some studies to contribute to increased chances of having a heart attack.
7. Other risk factors include sex, race, and age. Women are less likely to have heart attacks than men, perhaps because of protection from their hormonal system. However, after menopause the risk of heart attack in women begins to approach that of men. Blacks are more likely than whites to have high blood pressure and, therefore, a higher risk of heart attacks. And the older the individual, the more likely he or she is to have arteriosclerosis.

Signals of a Heart Attack

What is it like when a person develops a heart attack? The signals of a heart attack are usually obvious but vary from individual to individual. It is useful to understand the difference between a heart attack and an episode of angina. *Angina* is the term used to describe a temporary narrowing of a heart artery, which causes pain for several minutes but no permanent damage to the heart muscle. If the heart artery becomes completely blocked, then damage becomes permanent and a heart attack (myocardial infarction) has occurred.

Often patients who have a heart attack will have a history of angina. Angina is described as an uncomfortable pressure sensation, often characterized as squeezing, located in the center of the chest and radiating to the left arm, right arm, up into the neck or jaw, or even into the back. The pain is not usually described as sharp or stabbing. A patient with angina may experience some mild sweating, dizziness, or nausea. Should the pain continue for more than 10 minutes, then it is very likely that a heart attack has occurred.

The pain of a heart attack is more severe than angina and there is usually profuse sweating. Nausea and vomiting commonly occur. Shortness of breath is sometimes present and patients may feel dizzy. Patients who have heart attacks often have a sense of impending doom.

Many patients who have sudden cardiac arrest will have experienced symptoms of a heart attack prior to their collapse. However, it is important to appreciate that many patients who have sudden cardiac arrest will not have experienced symptoms of a heart attack prior to their collapse, and may have no symptoms whatsoever prior to their cardiac arrest. Even though they may have underlying heart disease as the cause of their cardiac arrest, they may not have experienced classic signs and symptoms of a myocardial infarction prior to collapse.

This chapter has focused on ventricular fibrillation due to underlying heart disease. However, ventricular fibrillation may occur in other settings, such as accidental electric shock, drownings, or intentional drug overdoses. An EMT encountering a patient without pulse or blood pressure in these settings must be aware of the possibility of ventricular fibrillation.

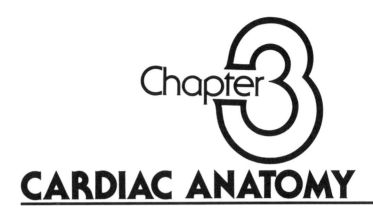

Chapter 3

CARDIAC ANATOMY

The Heart as a Pump

The heart is a muscle, and its major function is to pump blood throughout the body. The left side of the heart receives oxygenated blood from the lungs and pumps it through the arteries to all parts of the body. Blood that has delivered its oxygen to the cells of the body returns to the right side of the heart, which pumps it through the lungs, where carbon dioxide is given off and oxygen is absorbed. Then the process begins again with oxygenated blood returning to the left side of the heart. The heart has four chambers: two small atria and two large ventricles. The atria are the receiving chambers; they pump the blood into the two ventricles, which, in turn, have the major responsibility for pumping the blood to the lungs and body. Because the heart is a muscle, it must have its own supply of blood in order to contract repeatedly. The blood supply of the heart is carried by the coronary arteries. The coronary arteries, as they narrow with arteriosclerosis, may become completely blocked, resulting in the death of the heart muscle supplied by that artery.

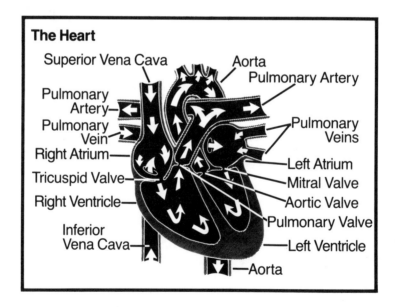

The Heart

Superior Vena Cava

Aorta

Pulmonary Artery

Pulmonary Artery

Pulmonary Vein

Right Atrium

Tricuspid Valve

Right Ventricle

Inferior Vena Cava

Pulmonary Veins

Left Atrium

Mitral Valve

Aortic Valve

Pulmonary Valve

Left Ventricle

Aorta

The Electrical System of the Heart

The heart is far more than just a muscle. Although any muscle has an electrical system that tells it when to contract, the cardiac muscle electrical system is a specialized system of interconnected cells spread throughout the entire heart. It provides and conducts the signal to the heart muscle to contract in a coordinated fashion. It is somewhat similar to the electrical wiring of a house. When the electrical system is turned on it causes the heart muscle fibers to contract. One electrical signal leads to one muscle contraction. The electrical impulse normally originates in a collection of electrical tissue called the *sinoatrial* (SA) node. The sinoatrial node receives its name because it is located in the sinus part of the atria. Impulses spread from the SA node in a wavelike fashion through both atria along internodal pathways located in the atrial muscle itself. The impulse then reaches a way station called the *atrioventricular* (AV) node. The atrioventricular node is so named because it is located between the atria and the ventricles. From the AV node the impulse enters the *bundle of His* and passes through left and right branches in the septum. The electrical impulse reaches the *Purkinje fibers,* located directly in the ventricular musculature, which in turn trigger the ventricular muscle to contract.

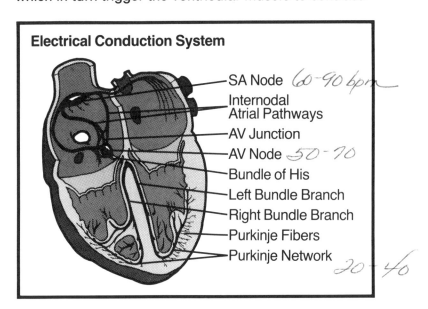

Electrical Conduction System

SA Node *60-90 bpm*
Internodal Atrial Pathways
AV Junction
AV Node *50-70*
Bundle of His
Left Bundle Branch
Right Bundle Branch
Purkinje Fibers
Purkinje Network *20-40*

SECONDARY PACEMAKERS

When everything works like it should, the SA node fires at approximately 60–100 beats per minute. The proper sequence is SA node to AV node to bundle of His to bundle branches to Purkinje fibers. Each time a firing sequence occurs, one coordinated contraction of the heart results. Although the SA node is normally the dominant pacemaker of the heart, any component of the conduction system can act as a secondary pacemaker should the SA node fail. The AV node, if it begins to act as the dominant pacemaker, usually fires at a rate of 40–50. The ventricular Purkinje fiber system, if it begins to act as the dominant pacemaker, fires at a rate of approximately 30–40 times per minute. The heart continues to beat automatically even if all nerve connections are severed or if the electrical conduction system is blocked. This characteristic is called *automaticity.* Usually the conduction system works in a very coordinated fashion. However, blocks or malfunctions can occur at any point along the pathway.

Working cells: need an electrical potential to work (nothing spontaneous)

electrical cells: have the capability to create action potential

Chapter 4

THE ELECTROCARDIOGRAM

For an EMT trained in the use of a defibrillator, it is not necessary to distinguish all the various cardiac rhythms. Clearly, the most important rhythm to recognize is ventricular fibrillation. However, the heart may have many normal and abnormal rhythms other than ventricular fibrillation. In order to understand the basic rhythms, it is necessary to appreciate how the electrocardiogram (ECG or EKG) works.

The electrocardiogram records an electrical picture of the heart's activity. The heart, as it contracts, releases small currents of electricity. These small currents are recorded by the electrocardiograph and the amplitude of each current is magnified. The deflections (movements above or below the baseline) are imprinted on heat sensitive paper or appear on an oscilloscope through deflection of a beam of electrons. When printed on paper rolling out of a machine at a constant rate, the result is the electrocardiogram.

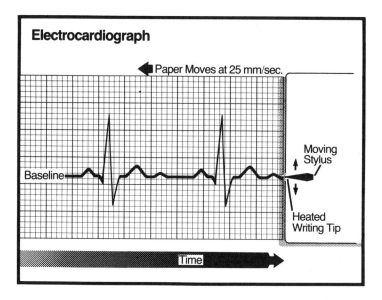

DEPOLARIZATION AND REPOLARIZATION

Each mechanical contraction of the heart (atria and ventricles) is associated with two electrical processes. The first is depolarization (activation), during which the electrical charges on the surface of the muscle change from positive to negative. The second process, repolarization, represents the return to a resting state, restoring positive surface charges on the heart muscle.

The electrocardiogram records the electrical forces produced by the heart. Since the body acts as a conductor of electrical current, any two points on the body may be connected with electrical leads. The resulting electrical activity of the heart is normally a series of regularly occurring waves and deflections on paper or oscilloscope.

Deflections of the ECG

The deflections of the ECG are arbitrarily labeled as the "P wave," the "QRS complex," and the "T wave."

P WAVE

The depolarization of the atria begins in the sinoatrial node. As the impulse exits from the SA node it causes depolarization of adjacent atrial muscle fibers, resulting in their contraction. The impulse continues to spread, radiating in wavelike forms across the two atria. The electrical signal passing through the atria produces the P wave.

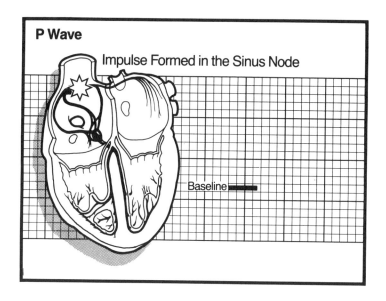

P Wave

Impulse Formed in the Sinus Node

Baseline

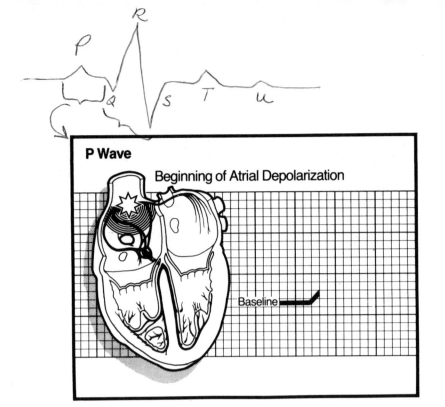

P Wave

Beginning of Atrial Depolarization

Baseline

P Wave

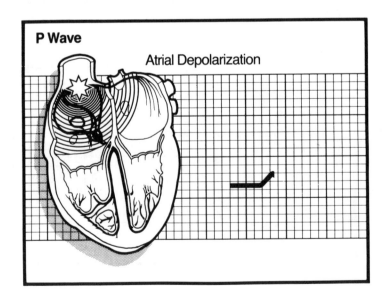

Atrial Depolarization

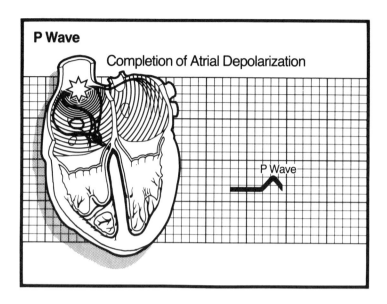

QRS COMPLEX

The wave then reaches the AV node, where the signal is transmitted down the bundle of His and into the ventricular muscle. As the signal is conducted along the electrical pathway, the QRS complex is produced.

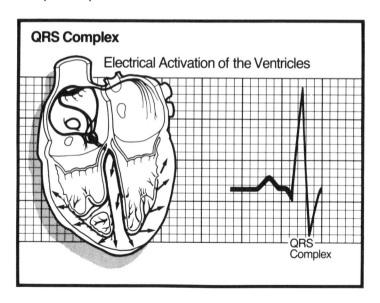

T WAVE

Following depolarization and contraction, the ventricles repolarize; restoration of electrical potential results in the T wave.

The complete cycle of P, QRS, and T represents one contrac-

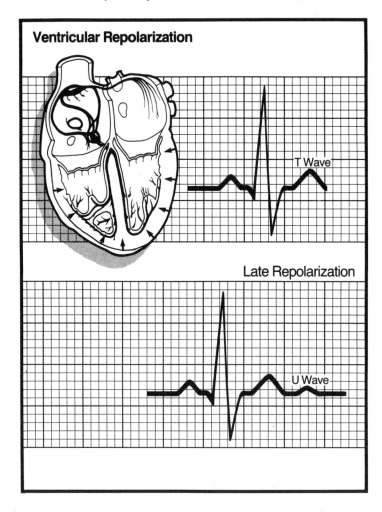

tion and repolarization of the heart muscle. It is important to realize that whether the deflection is upward or downward is a result of the position of the electrodes that are "reading" the electrical signal. By convention, the deflections of the P wave, QRS complex, and T wave are usually shown upright. However, the exact position (up or down) is of less importance than the proper sequence of P, QRS, and T.

Monitoring

An electrocardiogram is used to take multiple electrical pictures of the heart. Damage to various portions of the heart can then be determined. For EMT defibrillation, however, it is not necessary to take multiple pictures. It is only important to visualize the heart's rhythm with a single picture. This is called "monitoring." To monitor the rhythm, electrodes are appropriately attached to the patient's chest, usually with self-adhering, disposable disk electrodes. For usual monitoring purposes the positive electrode is placed near the left hip and the negative electrode near the right shoulder. This configuration is called a standard Lead II. The "ground" is usually placed near the left shoulder. If the defibrillator monitor being used has a switch to change leads it should always be on Lead II. Lead II is best for showing P waves and QRS complexes; therefore, although there are 12 possible leads, Lead II is the one most often used in prehospital care. Only Lead II will be shown in this book.

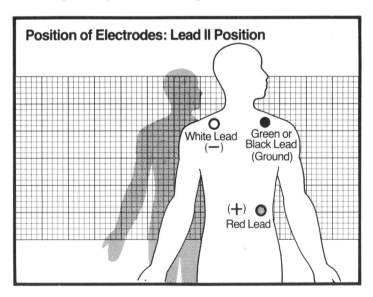

Position of Electrodes: Lead II Position

White Lead (−)

Green or Black Lead (Ground)

(+) Red Lead

ECG Paper

Electrocardiograms are recorded on specially marked graph paper used to measure amplitude and duration of the ECG signal. The paper is divided by light lines into 1 x 1mm squares and by dark lines into 5 x 5mm squares. Since the paper is moving at a speed of 25 mm per second, the light vertical lines represent .04 seconds

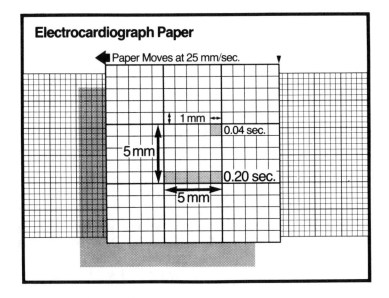

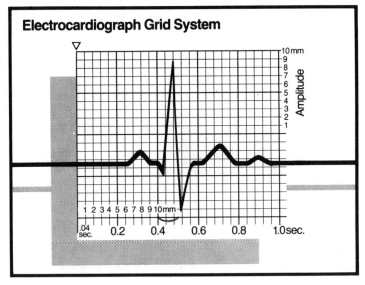

$P \longleftrightarrow R = 0.20$

$QRS = 0.12$

and the darker vertical lines represent 0.2 seconds. There are five dark lines per second. Markers at the top of the ECG paper are placed every three seconds.

Determining the Heart Rate

The heart rate may be calculated from the ECG strip by several methods. Using the six-second marker method, the QRS complexes present during a six-second interval are counted and multiplied by 10, resulting in the heart rate in beats per minute. Another method is the divisional method. The large squares between two QRS complexes are counted. This number is divided into 300. The result is the heart rate in beats per minute.

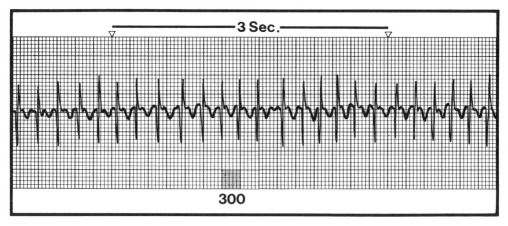

If the QRS complex occurs at every dark line, the rate is 300 per minute.

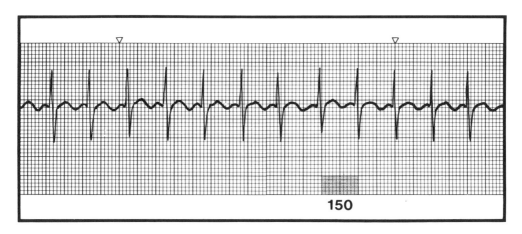

If there are two dark lines between complexes, rate is 150.

Three dark lines: 100.

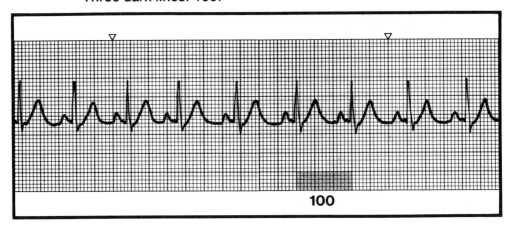

100

Four dark lines: 75.

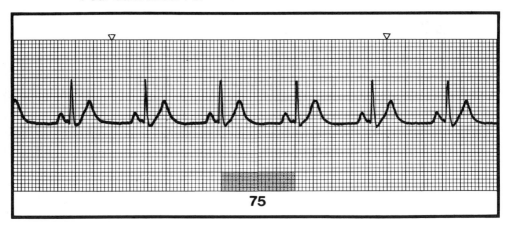

75

Five: 60. Six: 50.

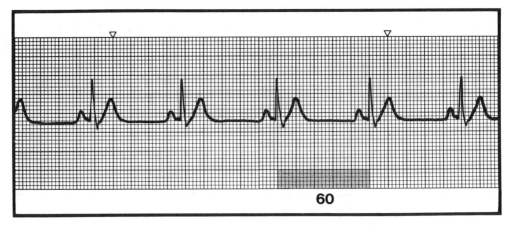

60

ECG Intervals

In addition to various deflections seen on the electrocardiogram, certain intervals are important. Since the paper is running at a fixed speed of 25 mm/second, it is possible to measure the interval between the various waves and deflections on the cardiogram.

The PR interval is the interval from the beginning of the P wave to the beginning of the QRS complex. It represents the time from the atrial depolarization to the beginning of ventricular depolarization. Normally, this time should not exceed 0.2 seconds, or one large square on ECG paper. The QRS complex represents the electrical depolarization of the ventricle, and its duration should not be greater than 0.12 seconds, or approximately half of a large box.

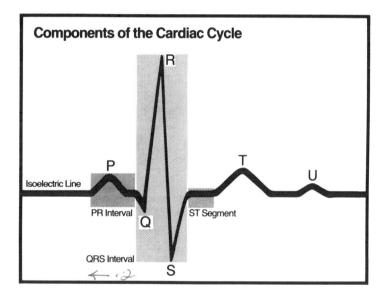

Components of the Cardiac Cycle

Pointers for Monitoring

It is important to remember the following points when monitoring patients:

1. A prominent P wave should be displayed if atrial activity is present.

2. If your defibrillator monitor has a rate meter, the QRS amplitudes should be sufficient to properly trigger it.

3. The chest of the patient should be left exposed so that defibrillation paddles can readily be applied if necessary.

4. It is important to remember that monitoring is for cardiac rhythm interpretation. It is impossible to tell whether there has been damage to the heart based only upon monitoring of the rhythm.

5. *Artifact* (extraneous mechanical or electrical interference with the ECG signal) should be noted and findings correlated with observations of the patient. For example: a straight line occurs if the patient cable is disconnected from the monitor.

A bizarre, wavey line resembling ventricular fibrillation may appear with faulty lead attachment.

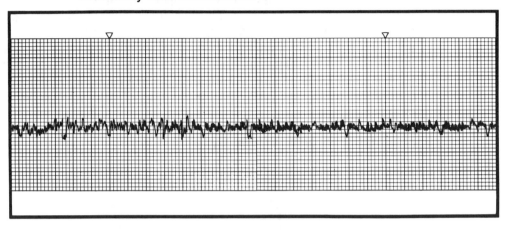

Artifact will also be caused by a patient's muscle tremors.

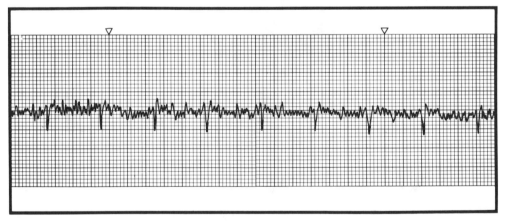

Sixty-cycle interference may be present if electrical appliances are in close proximity to the patient.

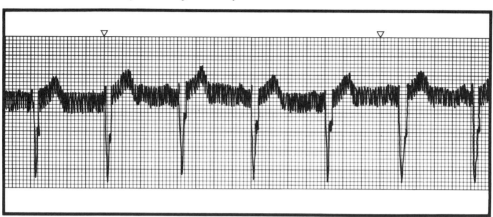

6. Causes of poor ECG signals may also include oily, dirty, or scaly skin; excessive hair; insufficient gel; or loose leads. Other causes are broken cable tips or wire and faulty grounding.

Rhythm Recognition

Recognizing the rhythm is of prime importance. The basic task is to distinguish ventricular fibrillation from other rhythms. In determining the rhythm, the following orderly steps should be taken:

1. Determine the heart rate. Heart rates less than 60 per minute are considered abnormally slow; heart rates greater than 100 per minute are considered abnormally fast. What is the atrial rate? What is the ventricular? Are they the same or different?

2. Analyze the cardiac rhythm. Is it regular (are P-to-R and R-to-R intervals constant)? If the rhythm is irregular, is it regularly irregular? That is, is the irregularity seen as a continuing pattern? Or is it irregularly irregular? That is, does the irregularity appear sporadically? Any abnormalities in the heart's conducting system will result in abnormalities in the ECG rhythm. Abnormalities may result from slowing of the electrical impulse through the heart, an abnormal focus initiating the electrical signal, or a complete blockage of the electrical signal at various points in the system. Variations in the shape and pattern of the ECG tracing result when signals are initiated from abnormal points, or blockages in the conducting system occur.

A pacemaker focus other than the SA node is known as an ectopic or out-of-place focus. Normally, there should be a P wave before every QRS complex. If P waves are not seen, it may be because the signal is not large enough to be seen on the rhythm strip, or because there is no atrial conduction. In such an instance, the ventricles may be contracting on their own. Generally, if the SA node fails to act as a pacemaker, either a different focus in the atria takes over or the impulse is initiated in the AV node.

When conduction through the atria or AV node is slowed, the PR interval becomes abnormally long. Initiation of electrical signals below the AV node alters the shape of the QRS complex. Generally, QRS complexes that are initiated from an abnormal location are widened, notched, or abnormally shaped.

Chapter 5

CARDIAC RHYTHMS

In this chapter the common normal and abnormal cardiac rhythms, including ventricular fibrillation, are discussed and illustrated.

Normal Sinus Rhythm

Normal sinus rhythm is the rhythm most commonly seen in healthy individuals. The rhythm originates in the sinoatrial node; thus the term "sinus."

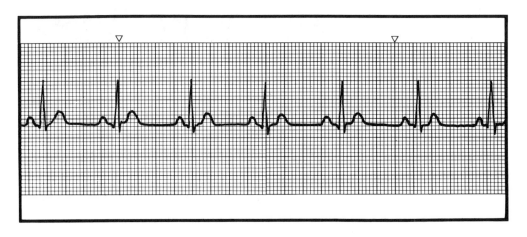

RECOGNITION

Rate: 60–100 beats per minute.

Rhythm: Regular.

Initiation of Electrical Activity: Electrical activity originates in the SA node.

CHARACTERISTIC FEATURES

P Waves: A P wave proceeds each QRS complex. The PR interval is less than 0.2 seconds.

QRS Complex: The QRS complex is tight, less than 0.12 seconds.

Normal Sinus Rhythm

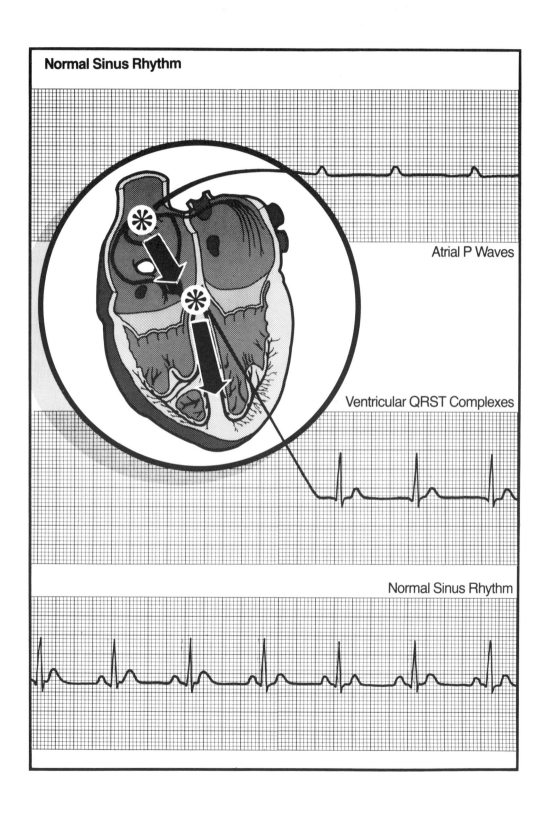

Atrial P Waves

Ventricular QRST Complexes

Normal Sinus Rhythm

Sinus Bradycardia

Sinus bradycardia is a slow heart rate. Electrical activity originates in the sinoatrial (SA) node. It looks just like normal sinus rhythm, except that the rate is less than 60 beats per minute. Sinus bradycardia may be seen normally in well-trained athletes. It is commonly found in individuals who have had an acute myocardial infarction. Although 50–60 can be tolerated, if the rate slows even more (40 or less) it is difficult to maintain a normal blood pressure. This is particularly true for elderly patients or patients with known heart disease. Patients with sinus bradycardia due to a suspected myocardial infarction require physician care as soon as possible.

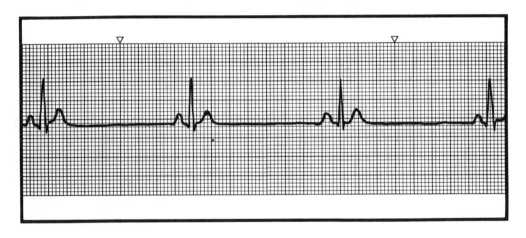

RECOGNITION

Rate: Less than 60.

Rythm: Regular

Initiation of Electrical Activity: Cardiac rhythm is initiated by the pacemaker in the SA node.

CHARACTERISTIC FEATURES:

P Wave and QRS Complex: P wave precedes each QRS complex. PR interval is less than 0.2 seconds, QRS complex is normally shaped and less than 0.12 seconds.

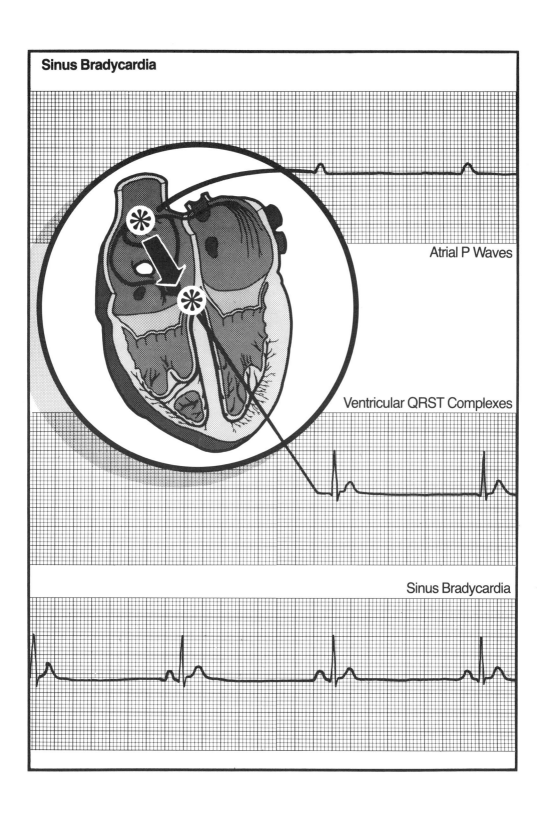

Sinus Bradycardia

Atrial P Waves

Ventricular QRST Complexes

Sinus Bradycardia

Sinus Arrhythmia

Sinus arrhythmia is a normal rhythm and refers to the periodic slowing and speeding up of the heart that is associated with respiratory activity. In some individuals (especially young adults) the heart rate slows with inspiration and speeds up with expiration.

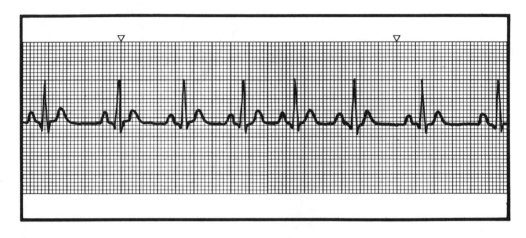

RECOGNITION

Rate: 60–100 per minute.

Rhythm: Irregular, slowing down and speeding up associated with inspiration and expiration.

Initiation of Electrical Activity: SA node.

CHARACTERISTIC FEATURES

P Wave and QRS Complex: A P wave precedes each QRS complex. The PR interval is less than 0.2 seconds. The QRS complex is normally shaped and less than 0.12 seconds.

Sinus Arrhythmia

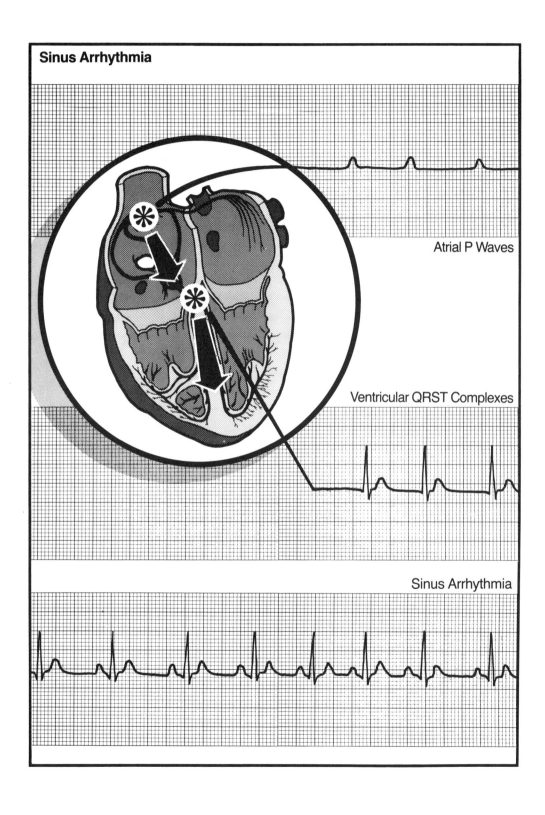

Atrial P Waves

Ventricular QRST Complexes

Sinus Arrhythmia

Sinus Tachycardia

Sinus tachycardia is a fast heart rate. Electrical activity is initiated in the sinoatrial node. Sinus tachycardia may be seen in a variety of conditions: exercise, fever, anxiety, and thyroid disease. In these conditions a fast heart rate is the normal bodily response to the needs for oxygen. Tachycardia may also be seen in heart disease; particularly in states of underoxygenation to the heart or as a result of damage to the heart. Therefore, tachycardia in the setting of chest pain (especially in an elderly person) may indicate the presence of myocardial infarction.

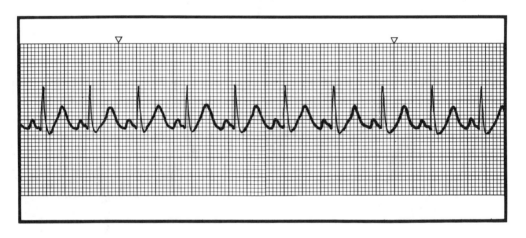

RECOGNITION

Rate: Greater than 100, usually less than 160.
Rhythm: Rhythm is regular.
Initiation of Electrical Activity: Occurs in the SA node.

CHARACTERISTIC FEATURES

P Waves: There is a P wave preceding each QRS complex. The P waves are sometimes buried in the preceding T wave and may not be distinct from the T wave.
QRS Complex: Tight, narrow, less than 0.12 seconds.

Sinus Tachycardia

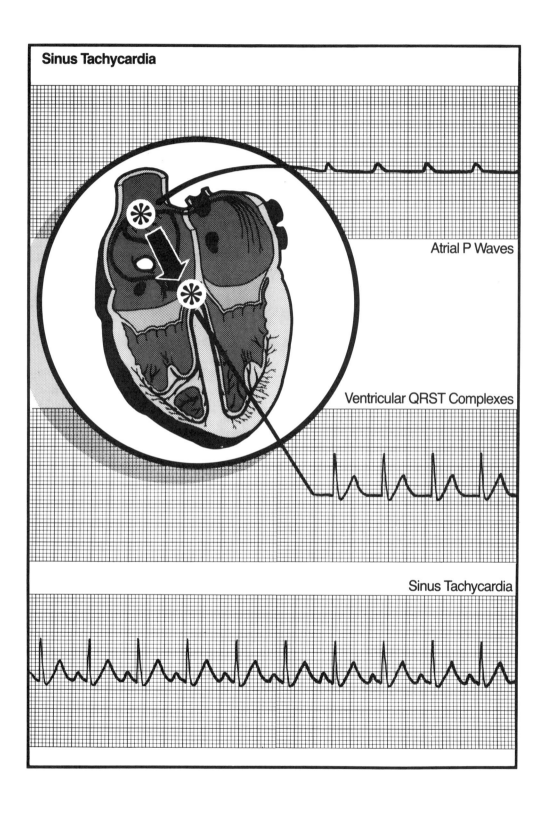

Atrial P Waves

Ventricular QRST Complexes

Sinus Tachycardia

Atrial Flutter

Impulse is coming from an area in the atrium

Atrial flutter is abnormal. As the name implies, it refers to fluttering of the atria. Fortunately, not all of the electrical waves from the atria are conducted into the ventricle; hence, the ventricle may still be contracting at a normal rate. The atria, in the state of flutter, beat at a rate of 240–350 per minute. Because the AV node acts as a "filter," only some of the beats get through to the ventricles. The ventricle rate is always slower and may be variable in nature. Generally, the ventricular rate is between 40 and 180 beats per minute. Atrial flutter often occurs in diseased hearts. It is often an unstable rhythm that commonly progresses to atrial fibrillation.

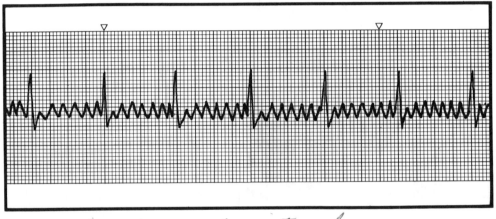

Usually regular intervals

RECOGNITION

Rate: The atria are beating at a rate of 240–350. Usually the ventricles are beating at a much slower rate of 40–180.

Rhythm: The rhythm of the QRS complexes may be regular or irregular.

Initiation of Electrical Activity: Electrical activity is initiated in the atrium at a location other than the SA node.

CHARACTERISTIC FEATURES

Flutter Waves (F): Often resemble a sawtooth pattern. They occur very rapidly; approximately one beat per large box of the ECG paper.

QRS Complex: Usually tight and narrow; occurs less often than the flutter waves (for example, every second or third or fourth flutter wave). This interval is not constant and may vary throughout time.

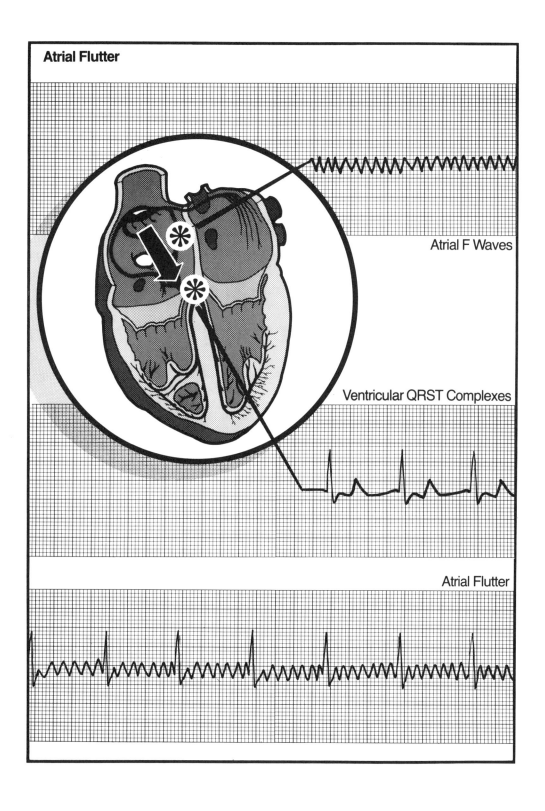

Atrial Flutter

Atrial F Waves

Ventricular QRST Complexes

Atrial Flutter

Atrial Fibrillation

Even though the term *atrial fibrillation* has "fibrillation" in its name, it is *not* ventricular fibrillation. It is completely different from ventricular fibrillation. Do not confuse atrial fibrillation with ventricular fibrillation. In atrial fibrillation, the atria beat chaotically but the ventricles are still beating in a coordinated fashion and blood pressure and pulse are maintained. Normal P waves are not observed. Instead there are very fine fibrillatory waves from the atria. Interspersed with these fine waves are the normal contractions of the ventricle.

Atrial fibrillation is an abnormal rhythm. However, people can live with this rhythm for many years. Hundreds of thousands, if not millions, of Americans have this rhythm. It is usually found in older individuals with underlying heart disease. As long as the ventricular rate remains in the normal range (60–100 per minute) these patients will not get into trouble. If, however, the ventricular rate becomes too fast, problems of hypotension or angina may result.

(Supraventricular tachycardia)

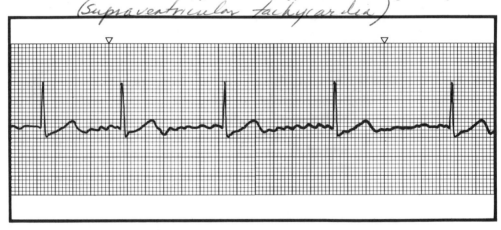

RECOGNITION

Rate: The atria are discharging at such a fast rate that distinct atrial waves cannot be counted. The rate is usually 400. The ventricular rate may vary from a low of 60 to a high of 160.

Rhythm: The rhythm is irregular. Specifically, the irregularity of the rhythm does not occur in a repeating pattern. Hence, the rhythm of atrial fibrillation is described as "irregularly irregular."

Initiation of Electrical Activity: Initial electrical activity occurs in the atria at many locations other than the SA node. The AV node acts as a "filter," and periodic signals are passed into the AV node for discharge of the ventricles.

CHARACTERISTIC FEATURES

Normal P waves are not present. Often, fine fibrillation waves (f) are seen between QRS complexes.

QRS Complex: Normal in configuration; occurs at irregularly irregular intervals. Rate of the ventricular contractions may range from 60 to 160.

Atrial Fibrillation

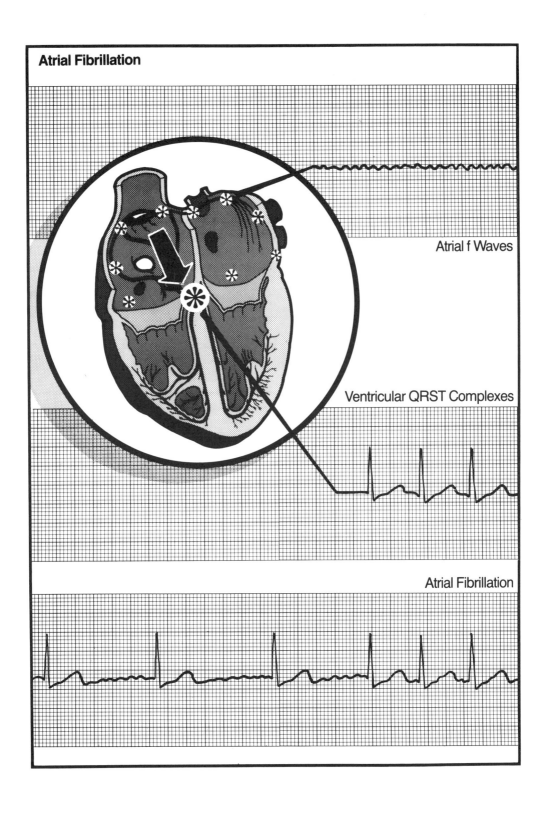

Atrial f Waves

Ventricular QRST Complexes

Atrial Fibrillation

Nodal Rhythm

In a nodal rhythm the electrical impulse is initiated at the AV node. The term *nodal* refers to the AV node and not the SA node. The SA node is quiet and there are no P waves seen. (Exceptions exist, but will not be covered here). Since the contraction is initiated in the AV node, the shape of the QRS is tight and normal in appearance. The rate may be slow or fast. Usually, but not always, nodal rhythms occur in the setting of acute myocardial infarction.

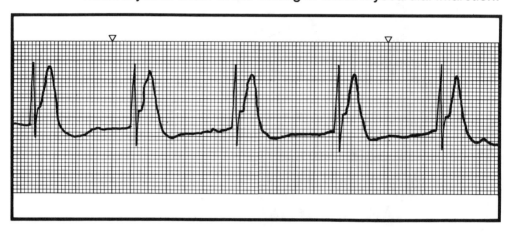

RECOGNITION

Rate: May be slow, normal, or fast.

Rhythm: Regular.

Initiation of Electrical Activity: Cardiac rhythm is initiated at the AV node.

CHARACTERISTIC FEATURES

P Waves: None present.

QRS Complex: Normal appearing, about 0.12 seconds or slightly greater in length.

Heart Blocks

Heart blocks are generally characterized as first degree, second degree, or third degree. Second-degree heart block has two types: Mobitz type I and Mobitz type II.

First-degree heart block. This block represents a prolongation of PR interval (greater than 0.20 seconds). This is not a dangerous rhythm and requires no specific treatment.

First Degree Heart Block

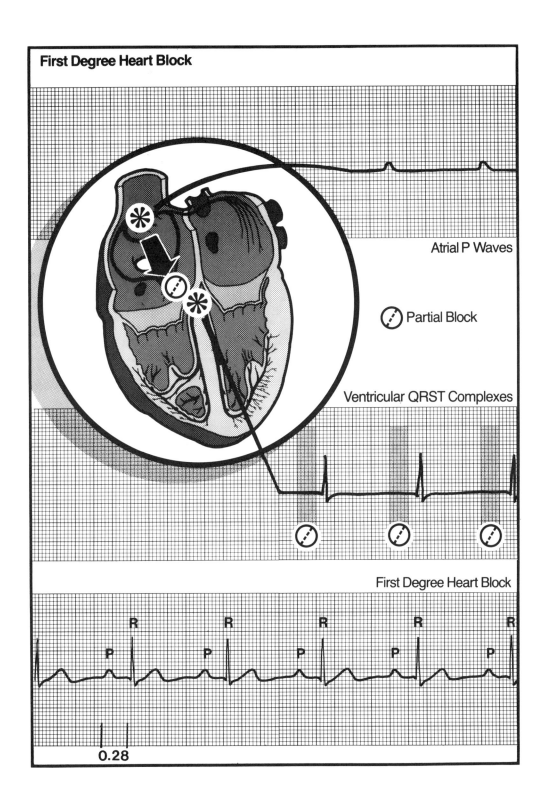

Atrial P Waves

Partial Block

Ventricular QRST Complexes

First Degree Heart Block

0.28

Second-degree heart block: Mobitz type I. This block represents a partial block through the AV node. There is a periodic dropped beat. In Mobitz type I the PR interval steadily lengthens until a beat or QRS complex is dropped. Mobitz type I may occur in acute myocardial infarction, but requires no specific treatment.

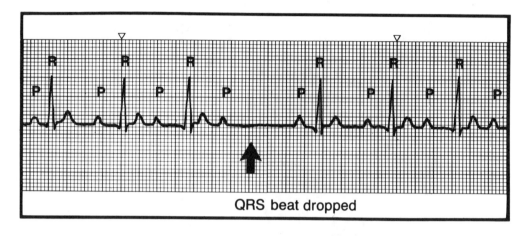

QRS beat dropped

Second-degree heart block: Mobitz type II. This block, which is more serious than Mobitz type I, represents a fixed block between the atria and the ventricles. Only one out of two, or one out of three, or one out of four atrial beats gets through to trigger the ventricles. The ventricular rate is often slow; patients may develop problems associated with this slow ventricular rate. It often occurs in the setting of acute myocardial infarction. This rhythm is serious and may progress to complete (third-degree) heart block.

Second Degree Heart Block – Mobitz Type II

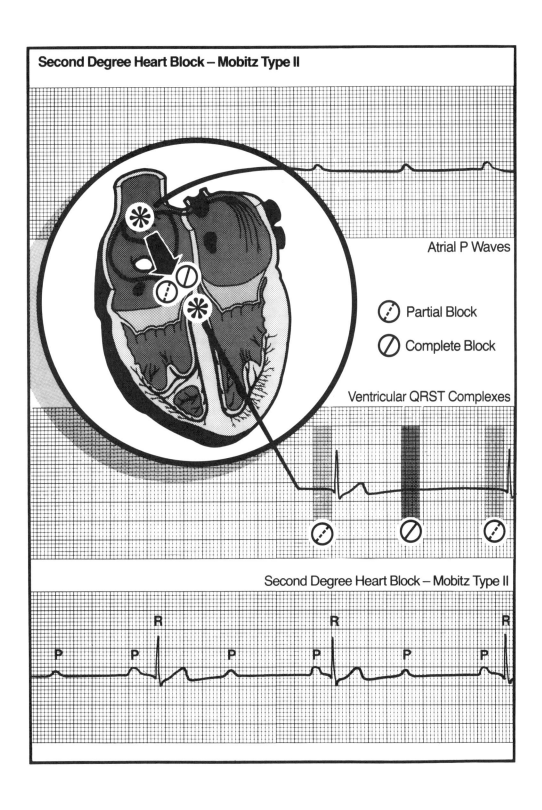

Atrial P Waves

Partial Block

Complete Block

Ventricular QRST Complexes

Second Degree Heart Block – Mobitz Type II

Third-degree heart block. This block is also known as complete heart block and is the most serious of heart blocks. It represents a complete separation of the atrial electrical signal from the ventricular electrical signal. Hence, no P waves are conducted through the AV node to trigger the ventricles. Because of this block, the AV node takes over and triggers the ventricles at a rate of approximately 40 beats per minute. This rhythm is very serious. It often occurs in the setting of an acute myocardial infarction and requires emergency drug medication or pacemaker therapy.

Recognizing the various heart blocks is not essential for the skill of EMT defibrillation, but general recognition is important, as people may be defibrillated into heart block.

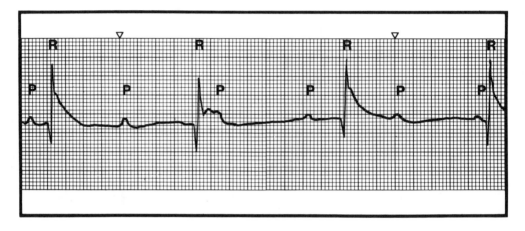

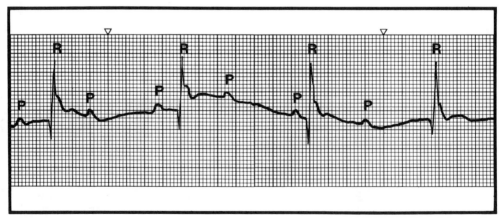

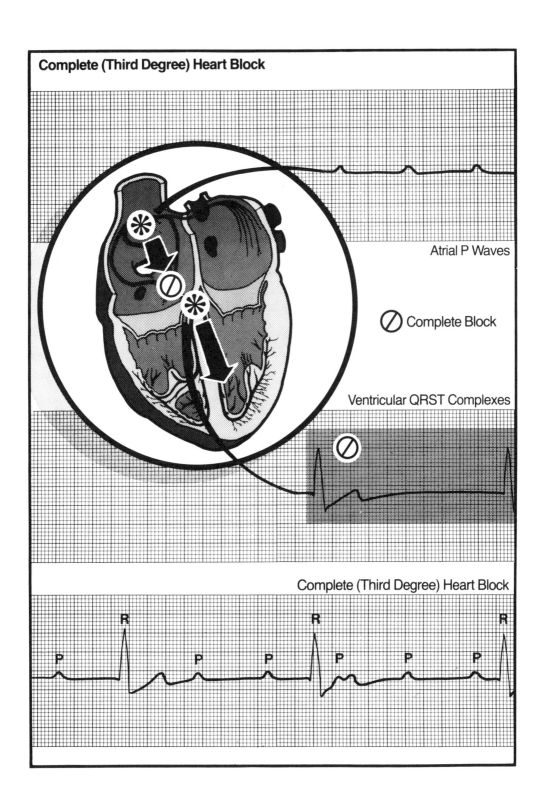

Complete (Third Degree) Heart Block

Atrial P Waves

⊘ Complete Block

Ventricular QRST Complexes

Complete (Third Degree) Heart Block

Premature Ventricular Contraction (PVC)

PVCs (or VPCs as they are also called) are extra electrical signals originating somewhere in the ventricle wall. This trigger point causes an abnormal contraction of the ventricular muscle. An occasional PVC by itself is not serious. However, it becomes serious in the setting of a diseased heart or an acute myocardial infarction. An individual with PVCs and chest pain due to a myocardial infarction is at very high risk for developing ventricular tachycardia or ventricular fibrillation. It is important to know that premature beats do not necessarily signify heart disease. However, PVCs in the setting of acute or sudden chest pain in an appropriately aged person are potentially dangerous.

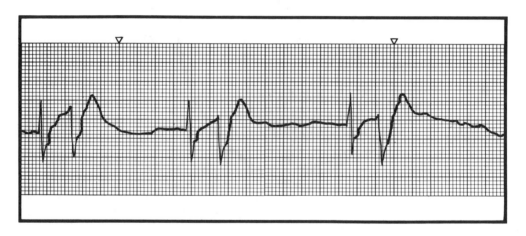

RECOGNITION

Rate: The rate is the underlying ventricular rate.

Rhythm: The rhythm is the underlying rhythm, but is irregular owing to the PVC, which occurs out of sequence. The underlying rhythm originates in the SA node.

Initiation of Electrical Activity: PVCs occur somewhere in the periphery of the ventrical wall. They do not originate in the AV node.

CHARACTERISTIC FEATURES

P Wave and QRS Complex: There is no P wave preceding the *premature* contraction. The contraction is abnormal in shape when compared to the normal QRS complex. It is greater than 0.12 seconds in length. T waves of the premature contraction are directed opposite to the normal T wave. If two or more premature ventricular contractions occur together, they are *couplets.*

The big wide beat s̄ a P wave due to the slower impulse from ventricles

MULTIFOCAL PVCs

If two premature contraction have different configurations, they have different points of origin and are referred to as *multifocal PVCs.* Multifocal PVCs are ominous. The patient with multifocal PVCs is at great risk of developing ventricular fibrillation or ventricular tachycardia. By definition, three or more PVCs in a row are considered ventricular tachycardia.

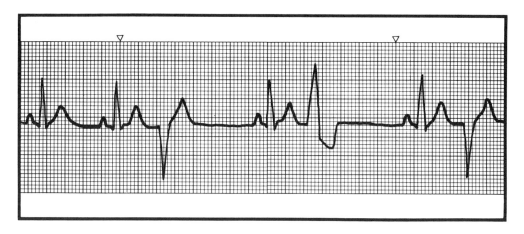

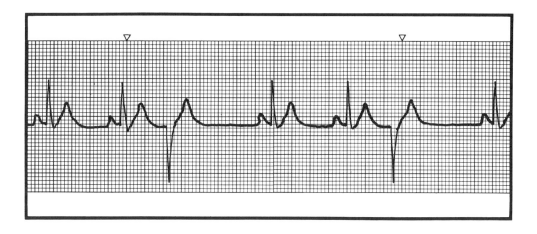

Normal beats can be coupled with PVCs. When a pattern of normal beats and PVCs is established, this is called *bigeminy.* A pattern of two normal beats with a PVC is called *trigeminy.*

Ventricular Tachycardia

Ventricular tachycardia is life-threatening and must be treated rapidly if the patient is to survive. Patients with good heart function can tolerate ventricular tachycardia for a period of time ranging from minutes sometimes even to hours. Elderly persons with marginal heart function tolerate ventricular tachycardia for only a short period of time; in just seconds or minutes, the ventricular tachycardia will deteriorate to ventricular fibrillation. The most common setting for the occurrence of ventricular tachycardia is acute myocardial infarction.

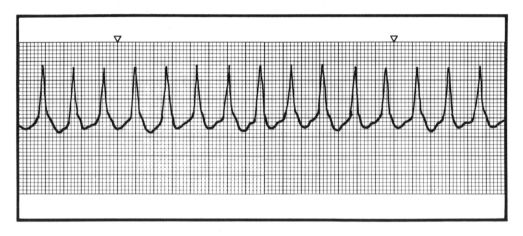

RECOGNITION

Rate: Usually 140–200 beats per minute.

Rhythm: Rhythm is almost regular.

Initiation of Electrical Activity: electrical activity is initiated from an ectopic focus in the ventricles. This supresses the normal electrical activity of the heart.

CHARACTERISTIC FEATURES

P Waves: None seen.

QRS Complexes: Wide, slurred, abnormally shaped, longer than 0.12 seconds.

NOTE: *The patient's vital signs deteriorate rapidly in the setting of ventricular tachycardia.*

Ventricular Tachycardia

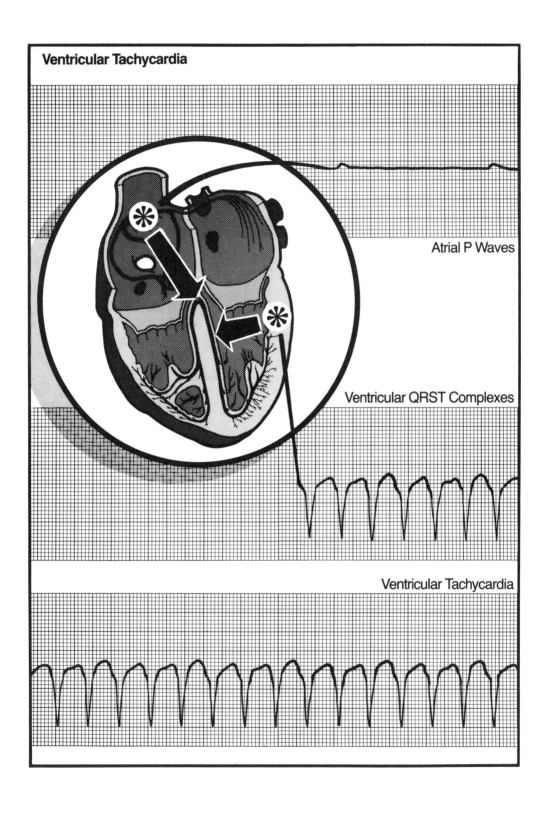

Atrial P Waves

Ventricular QRST Complexes

Ventricular Tachycardia

Ventricular Flutter

*doesn't last long →
converts to fib.*

Ventricular flutter is a transition arrhythmia that occurs when ventricular tachycardia degenerates into ventricular fibrillation. Ventricular flutter last only seconds. There is no pulse or blood pressure. An EMT should prepare for defibrillation, as the rhythm will become ventricular fibrillation by the time the paddles have been charged.

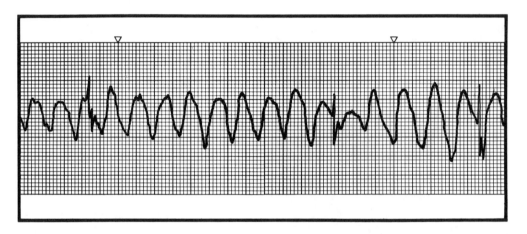

Ventricular Fibrillation

Ventricular fibrillation is the rhythm that, when recognized, can be treated by an EMT with a defibrillator. Ventricular fibrillation is fatal unless treated with an electric shock. A defibrillatory shock delivered to a fibrillating heart can produce a normally beating heart. A patient in ventricular fibrillation has no pulse or blood pressure and is unconscious. *It is impossible for the patient to be in ventricular fibrillation and talk to you.*

Ventricular fibrillation can occur in the setting of myocardial infarction. It can also occur without any warning whatsoever.

With proper training and experience, the EMT can distinguish ventricular fibrillation from all other rhythms. IT HAS A CHARACTERISTIC, CHAOTIC PATTERN TOTALLY UNLIKE ANY OTHER RHYTHM. The fibrillatory waves result from firing sites in the ventricles. The ventricles are firing in such a rapid, chaotic pattern that no blood can be propelled from the heart. It is for this reason that the pulse is zero and the blood pressure falls to zero.

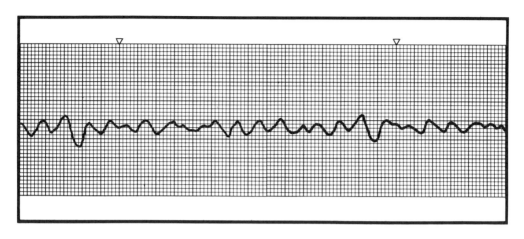

RECOGNITION

Rate: Indeterminate because of the multiple chaotic pattern and lack of QRS complexes.

Rhythm: Totally irregular; no repeating pattern whatsoever.

Initiation of Electrical Activity: Multiple sites throughout the ventricles initiate the fibrillatory waves.

CHARACTERISTIC FEATURES

The pattern is completely chaotic. There is no organized electrical pattern.

TREATMENT FOR VENTRICULAR FIBRILLATION

A defibrillatory shock is to be administered as rapidly as possible. The only ECG patterns that can be mistaken for ventricular fibrillation are artifact due to muscle movement by the patient, and interpretation mistakes because of inappropriate calibration of the monitor. When determining the rhythm, be absolutely certain that the patient is not being moved and that there is no obvious muscle activity (*i.e.,* shivering). If the machine has been properly calibrated prior to arrival the likelihood of misinterpretation of the rhythm is negligible.

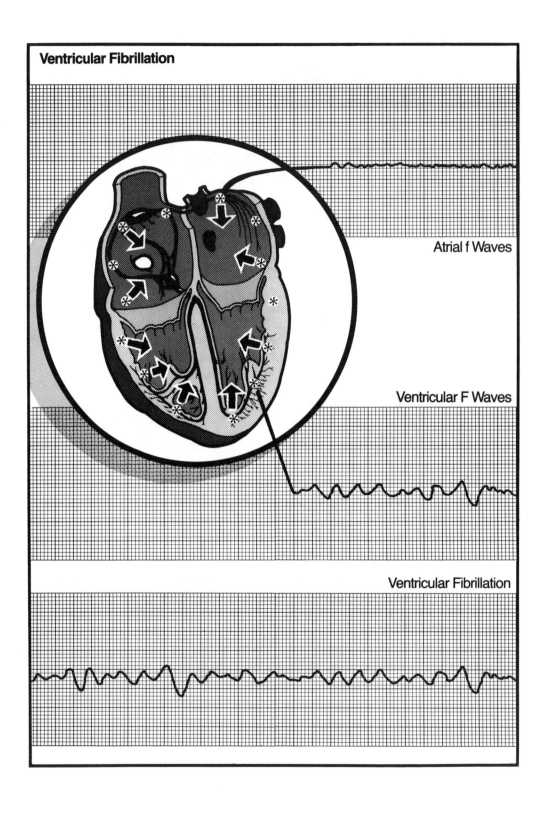

Ventricular Fibrillation

Atrial f Waves

Ventricular F Waves

Ventricular Fibrillation

Fine Ventricular Fibrillation

Fine ventricular fibrillation is identical to regular (coarse) ventricular fibrillation except that the amplitude of the fibrillatory waves is not as great. Fine ventricular fibrillation probably occurs after the heart has been in ventricular fibrillation for several minutes. Usually "coarse" ventricular fibrillation gradually (over 5–10 minutes) weakens into "fine" ventricular fibrillation. There is no specific demarcation between "coarse" and "fine" ventricular fibrillation; these are not two distinct rhythms. Hearts in fine ventricular fibrillation are more difficult to defibrillate. The coarser the ventricular fibrillatory pattern, the more likely it is that the rhythm will respond to electric defibrillatory shocks. Fine ventricular fibrillation may appear because of undercalibration of the monitor. Whenever ventricular fibrillation is encountered, be it fine or coarse, the treatment is defibrillatory shock.

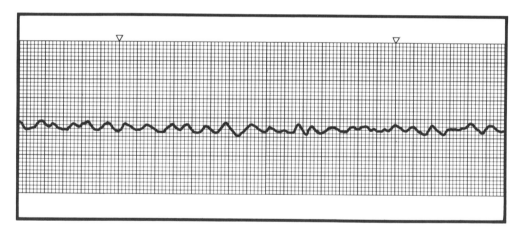

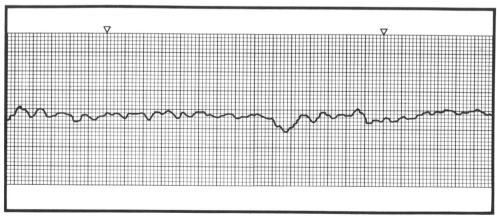

Idioventricular Rhythm

Idioventricular rhythm is a critical situation. Individuals in this rhythm are IN CARDIAC ARREST. The patient is without pulse or blood pressure. This rhythm is different from ventricular fibrillation. It is a very slow rate. The electrical signal is ventricular and is initiated at a focus other than the AV node. In idioventricular rhythm, the heart is dying. The usual setting is cardiac arrest as a result of myocardial infarction.

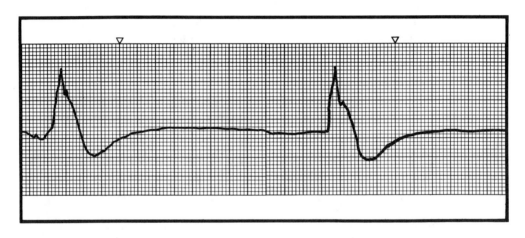

RECOGNITION
Rate: Very slow; less than 20 per minute.
Rhythm: May be regular or irregularly slow.
Initiation of Electrical Activity: From an ectopic focus in the ventricle.

CHARACTERISTIC FEATURES
P Waves: None present.
QRS Complex: Wide and bizarre appearing. Very, very slow rate with an ineffective contraction of the heart, so that a pulse or blood pressure is usually not maintained.

Asystole

In asystole, there is no electrical activity in the heart. It is a flat line rhythm and is present when the heart is dead. Asystole may occur as the end point of ventricular fibrillation. It may also occur as a result of a massive myocardial infarction. Defibrillation has no effect on asystole. Occasionally, medications may stimulate asystole into some sort of electrical activity.

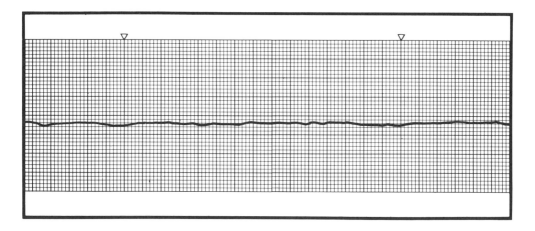

Chapter 6

DEFIBRILLATION

Modern defibrillators were developed in the 1960s. However, experimentation with electrical defibrillation occurred as early as 1890. The first published account of a successful animal defibrillation occurred in 1933, and the first human defibrillation in 1947. Early defibrillators utilized 60 hertz alternating current or 60 cycle. It was found soon after introduction of AC defibrillators that direct current (DC) defibrillators produced a more effective wave form with fewer side effects. All defibrillators on the market today use DC current.

Defibrillation, put simply, is the delivery of an electric current through the chest wall and heart for the purpose of terminating ventricular fibrillation. In ventricular fibrillation, the electrical system within the heart muscle is chaotically firing hundreds of signals per minute, resulting in a totally ineffective heart. As no blood is being expelled, blood pressure immediately falls to zero and the pulse immediately disappears. Delivery of a large jolt of electricity through the heart depolarizes all of the cells at once so the heart's normal pacemaker may resume firing in an orderly fashion.

Design of the Defibrillator

The DC defibrillator is constructed so that the paddle electrodes can deliver electricity directly through the chest wall and into the heart. Portable defibrillators employed in prehospital emergency care utilize batteries to store power. Upon the charging of the defibrillator, energy travels from the battery to the capacitor. Once

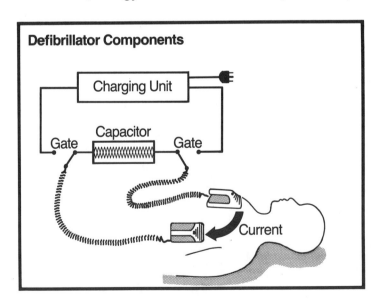

Defibrillator Components

Charging Unit

Capacitor

Gate   Gate

Current

the capacitor is fully charged, if the current is released into the patient, energy travels from one paddle through the patient's chest to the other paddle. When the capacitor is charging, the current does not flow through the paddles into the patient. However, during discharge, the circuit swings open from the capacitor, allowing electricity through the cables and into the paddles. Charging of the paddles generally takes 10–15 seconds. Discharge occurs, however, in a very short time (usually 5–30 milliseconds) once the discharge buttons are depressed. Storage of the charge can only be maintained for a short period, as "bleeding down" of energy of the charge will occur. The "bleeding down" will typically occur over 30 seconds, depleting 70–90% of the initial charge.

ENERGY: STORED AND DELIVERED

Energy is measured in joules. Joules were formerly called "watt seconds" and older machines may still indicate energy in watt seconds. Some machines measure energy in terms of stored energy; others measure in terms of delivered energy. Generally, delivered energy is approximately 80% of stored energy. (The falloff in energy is the result of losses within the circuitry of the defibrillator as well as resistance to the flow of current across the chest wall.) Since the delivered energy depends to some extent upon the size of the patient and skin resistance, it is important to realize that statements about delivered energy are only approximations. A rough rule of thumb is to take 80% of stored energy to approximate the amount of joules delivered to the patient.

CONTROLS

For simplicity and ease of operation, most modern defibrillators have a limited number of controls. Generally there is a power switch, an energy select control, a charge control, and two discharge buttons (usually placed on the paddles). An EMT must familiarize him/herself with the particular machine used in his/her emergency agency.

PADDLES

Paddles are often designated as to location of use, such as "apex" or "sternum." Place the "sternum" paddle on the right side of the patient's chest lateral to the upper sternum and below the right clavicle. Place the "apex" paddle on the lower left side of the patient's chest, below and lateral to the apex of the heart. If your defibrillator is equipped with "QUIK-LOOK®" capability, placing the paddle in the proper location is important for standardized reading of the electric signal of the heart. However, the signal can still be read if the paddles are reversed; ECG deflection will simply be downward instead of upward. Adequate defibrillation will occur whether the apex paddle is in the apex or in the sternum position and whether the sternum paddle is in the sternum location or at the apex.

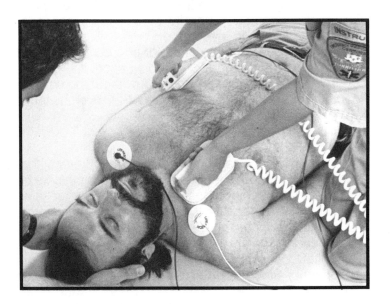

Other Uses of a Defibrillator

Most modern defibrillators are also able to provide synchronized cardioversion. Synchronized cardioversion is not used in EMT defibrillation programs. However, since the capability for cardioversion is built into most defibrillators, a few words are in order.

Synchronized cardioversion is utilized for abnormally fast heart rhythms in order to interrupt the ectopic pacemaker and allow the normal SA node to regain command of the heart's rhythm. This procedure is only used on rhythms that have organized QRS complexes. The word *synchronized* refers to the fact that the shock is delivered at a specific point in the cardiac cycle. When the defibrillator is in the synchronized mode, it recognizes the QRS complex and delivers the charge 10 milliseconds after the QRS complex is sensed.

The synchronized mode must never be used for defibrillating ventricular fibrillation. If the synchronized mode is inadvertently turned on, the defibrillator will not deliver a defibrillatory shock, since there are no QRS complexes in ventricular fibrillation.

Unless specifically authorized by the program Medical Director, EMTs are not to employ synchronized cardioversion.

Energy Requirements

The proper amount of joules delivered to the patient should be enough to depolarize the heart cells but not so much that damage to the cardiac muscle occurs. There has been controversy in recent years regarding high-energy *versus* low-energy defibrillatory shocks for ventricular fibrillation. A recent study suggested that low energy (175 joules) is just as effective as higher energy (330 joules) and is less likely to cause cardiac damage or postshock abnormal rhythms. Given the, as yet, lack of agreement about the best energy level, we recommend using an intermediate level of 200 joules (delivered energy). This level of energy is consistent with American Heart Association Advanced Cardiac Life Support Guidelines. It is important to know whether your machine lists stored or delivered energy, since the recommendation of 200 joules is *delivered* energy. If your machine lists *stored* energy the amount should be about 250 joules. If the settings on your machine are not calibrated at this exact energy level, use the closest higher level. In other words, if your machine has a setting of 225 instead of 200 utilize the energy setting 225.

Some machines are available that can deliver very high amounts of energy (greater than 400 joules). We do not recommend energy levels above 400 joules except under physician or paramedic supervision.

We realize that the "correct" amount of energy necessary for safe defibrillation has not been sufficiently studied in humans. Hence, our recommendations are only guidelines, and local practices should be followed. Furthermore, as more information becomes available these guidelines may change.

Energy requirements for pediatric defibrillation are less than those for adults, for the obvious reason of a smaller body mass. Dosage recommendation is one joule per pound of weight. Ventricular fibrillation in children is very rare, and unless specifically authorized by the Medical Director, we do not recommend defibrillation for children under 12.

Sequence of Defibrillation

1. Lubricate paddles with conductive gel. Enough gel should be used to cover the surface of the paddles, but not so much as to slop over the sides.

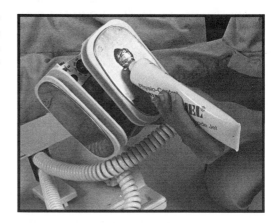

2. Turn the defibrillator power on and select the energy level (200 joules).

3. Be certain that the defibrillator is not in the synchronous mode.

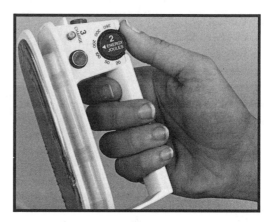

4. Charge defibrillator.

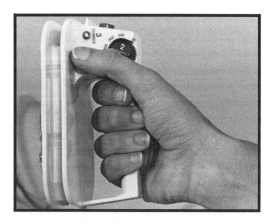

5. Place paddles on patient's bare chest. Firm pressure should be used (approximately 25 pounds) in order to have good contact between the paddle electrodes and the patient's skin. When placing the paddles and using gel, do not allow the gel to bridge the two paddle sites, as the delivered energy may arc along the surface of the skin.

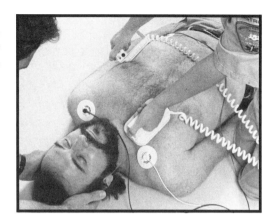

6. Make certain no one is touching the patient's bed or any metal object connected to the patient. Shout "CLEAR" before discharging the paddles.

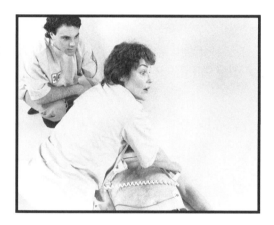

7. Depress both paddle buttons simultaneously. If the charge has been delivered, patient may give a muscle-jerk response unless downtime is excessive.

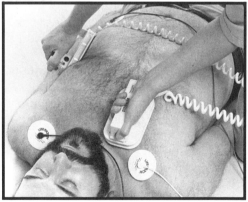

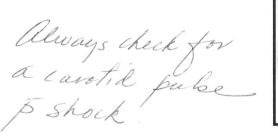

Always check for a carotid pulse p̄ shock!

8. Assess the post shock rhythm, taking no longer than 15 seconds. If a delay of 15 seconds or more is encountered due to battery problems, artifact, uncertainty of rhythm, etc., resume CPR until the problem is resolved and then reassess."

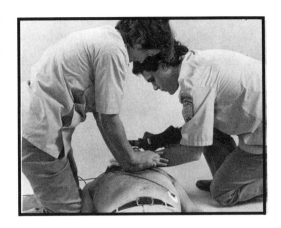

9. If the patient remains in ventricular fibrillation, a second defibrillatory shock of 200 joules may be given, followed by up to 30 seconds of CPR, then reassess the rhythm.

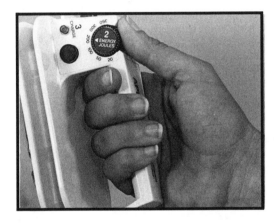

10. If ventricular fibrillation still remains, a third defibrillatory shock of 200 joules may be given, followed by up to 30 seconds.

NOTE: *Some local protocols will call for an increase to 300–360 joules for the third attempt. Whether this is done or not is determined by the controlling medical authority.*

We believe that three shocks is the maximum number to be delivered. If three shocks have not defibrillated the heart it is unlikely that additional shocks will be of benefit; they may only deprive the patient of necessary CPR. If ventricular fibrillation persists the patient needs emergency medications and correction of acidosis. This can on-

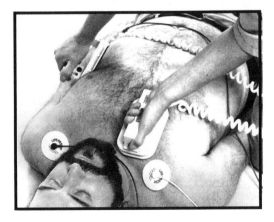

ly be provided by paramedics of physicians. Hence, if three shocks have not been sufficient, the EMT must continue CPR and either await paramedic arrival (assuming such personnel and services are available) or transport the patient with ongoing CPR to the hospital. If, however, the third defibrillatory shock produced a *perfusing rhythm* and after a period of time the patient goes back into ventricular fibrillation, *one* more defibrillatory shock may be given according to the procedures outlined above.

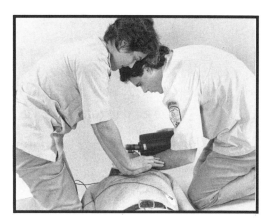

Another type of defibrillator will defibrillate automatically. Electrodes on the chest sense when ventricular fibrillation is occurring and the machine automatically delivers the necessary electric energy. This type of defibrillator is a recent development, and as the technology improves it may have field application. However, as with any technology, it does not replace the need for knowledge and judgment.

Maintenance of Equipment

The defibrillator is an expensive, precision medical instrument. To insure that it will be operational at all times, ongoing daily maintenance of the machine is required. A standardized check-off procedure should be established for the particular defibrillator purchased. The following maintenance should be performed routinely:

1. **Check the battery.** Be certain that the batteries are freshly charged. The level of battery charge should be checked at least daily and a routine established for rotation of batteries. Nickel cadmium (NiCad) batteries are commonly used in portable defibrillators. A problem with these batteries is the acquisition of "memory". Unless the batteries are used so that their energy is drained down and then recharged again, they will not completely store a charge. In other words, if they are only allowed to drain down slightly and then recharged again, over and over, "memory" will build up in the battery and the available power following recharging will be considerably shortened. Therefore, you need to

purchase a battery discharger and run the battery all the way down before recharging.

2. Check the operation of the defibrillator itself. There are several methods of testing defibrillator operation; follow the recommendations for your particular equipment. Defibrillators should not be tested by open-air discharge, as discharging the paddles into the air can result in an inadvertent jolt to the operator. Another test that is not recommended is to place the two paddles face-to-face. While this may not harm the operator, it can easily pit the paddle surface, which can impair the ability of the paddles to deliver energy effectively into the patient's skin.

Defibrillators can reliably be tested with a defibrillator tester, which in some machines is built into the unit and in others requires a separate piece of equipment. Testers have metal plates or contacts for the paddles and a discharge switch that, when activated, indicates that energy has been discharged.

3. Check paper and stylus. Many defibrillators are sold with ECG paper printout capability. Machines with ECG paper recorders should be checked to determine whether the stylus is properly recording. A fresh supply of paper should always be in place.

Calibration

Most defibrillator monitors on the market have the means to calibrate the monitor. Calibration refers to the proper adjustment of the electric signal into the monitor. When a machine is properly calibrated, a fixed amount of electricity will result in a standardized deflection on the oscilloscope or ECG paper. By convention, one millivolt of electricity should result in a deflection of one centimeter (two large squares of ECG paper, or approximately ½ inch). When the calibration button is pressed, one millivolt is amplified onto the oscilloscope. Calibration should be adjusted so that this energy results in the proper deflection of one cm. Calibration is very important because if the machine is undercalibrated or overcalibrated a wrong interpretation of the cardiac rhythm may be made. For example, if the machine is undercalibrated, the patient's ECG signal will appear smaller than it really is. A patient who is *really* in ventricular fibrillation may appear to be in asystole. Obviously, such a mistake would result in a shock not being given when it should be. On the other hand, if the machine is overcalibrated, the ECG signal will be overly magnified. Thus, what really is asystole may appear to be ventricular fibrillation, resulting in the patient's being shocked when no shock is indicated. Also, overcalibration will increase the amount of artifact and make the rhythm more difficult to interpret. Hence, proper calibration is exceedingly important. It is the only way to assure that what you see on the monitor is what the patient really has.

Safety

It is essential that safe procedures be followed at all times. The defibrillator, if used improperly, can inadvertently shock the operator or other emergency personnel at the scene. While such a shock may only stun the individual, it does have the potential to kill. A defibrillatory shock, inappropriately delivered to a heart that is beating normally, may jolt the heart into the rhythm of ventricular fibrillation. Obviously, such an occurrence is to be avoided. The only way to avoid such a calamity is to be extremely careful. The following precautions should be taken at all times:

1. The operator should be certain that all emergency personnel are clear of the patient or bed prior to defibrillation. Shout "CLEAR" prior to pressing the two paddle buttons, and see that everyone is out of danger.
2. Do not touch the patient while defibrillating; touch only the handles on the paddles.
3. Do not use excessive gel, which may goop over the sides of the defibrillator paddles and touch the operator's knuckles. Too much gel may also bridge across the patient's chest wall and cause a spark or bridging of the electricity.
4. Do not dump the load through open-air discharge or paddle-to-paddle placement if it is decided not to deliver the energy. Dump the load according to the recommendations of the manufacturer.
5. Clean the paddles after use. Dried gel can continue to conduct electricity and may cake up on the side of the defibrillator paddle handle.
6. Do not have the person performing CPR, whose hands may become coated with gel, take over and operate the defibrillator paddles. The gel on his hands may conduct the electric charge.

Is it safe to defibrillate in the rain? Generally it is. However, if possible, the chest should be wiped dry between the defibrillator paddle sites. Rain water does not conduct electricity well, but the conductive gel may dissolve in the rain water and spread across the chest wall. Keep your hands as dry as possible when operating a defibrillator in the rain.

Is it safe to defibrillate on a metal deck? Generally it is, so long as the paddles are placed in the proper position and do not touch the metal flooring. Be extra careful not to touch the patient at the time of discharge.

Troubleshooting

The EMT should be aware of some common problems associated with defibrillation. The most common problem is inadvertently dumping the load prior to discharge. As mentioned above, most machines "bleed down" their charge and may require recharging prior to delivery of the defibrillatory shock.

Inadvertently pressing the "POWER" button on the defibrillator paddles when the unit is already on and charged is a common problem. This action will disarm the defibrillator and require that the power and charge control be reactivated. Only some machines have the charging button located on the paddle.

A third problem is not pressing the two discharge buttons simultaneously.

Another problem is inadvertently pressing the synchronous-mode button found on some defibrillators. If this button is pressed the defibrillator will not discharge for ventricular fibrillation. Turn off the synchronous switch and try again.

If an attempted defibrillation is made and the patient does not have a jerk response, it is possible that the electric shock was not delivered. The EMT should rapidly find the reason, recharge the paddles, and deliver the defibrillatory shock.

Chapter 7

SAVING A LIFE

Defibrillation Protocol

The skills required for EMT defibrillation are easy to master. With adequate preparation and practice, EMTs will undoubtedly have the opportunity to attempt defibrillation for patients in ventricular fibrillation and may indeed save a life.

The most important step is to confirm that cardiac arrest is present. This is done in the standard fashion, with rapid assessment of airway, breathing, and circulation. Standard practice should be followed: "shake and shout"; open the airway; look, listen, and feel for 10 seconds to detect respirations; deliver four stacked ventilations followed by a 5–10 second determination of the carotid pulse. If the carotid pulse is not present, then chest compression is to be initiated. Depending upon personnel available, this can be one-person or two-person CPR. If only two EMTs are at the scene, one-person CPR should be initiated while the other EMT trained to defibrillate attaches the monitor leads.

The EMT responsible for the machine should turn it on and immediately identify the situation (*see* Documenting the Event, p. 76). Assuming the defibrillator has a cassette recorder, the EMT should identify him or herself, describe the sex and approximate age of the patient, and verbally describe what is happening. At this time it is appropriate to run a paper strip to document the patient's cardiac rhythm.

1. Take adequate time (at least six seconds) to look at the cardiac rhythm. This is about two sweeps on most cardioscopes. No longer than 10 seconds should be taken to identify the rhythm.
2. If ventricular fibrillation is present, gel the paddles and charge them to 200 joules.
3. Stop CPR, assess the rhythm one last time as a safety check, and deliver the first countershock.
4. After delivery of the first shock assess the post shock rhythm taking no longer than 15 seconds. If QRS complexes are seen, determine whether they result in a pulse; if a pulse is present, then determine the blood pressure. If no pulse or blood pressure is present, then of course CPR must be resumed.

If the patient remains in ventricular fibrillation after the first countershock, a second shock may be delivered observing the same sequence. Determine the rhythm while CPR is stopped. If ventricular fibrillation is present, deliver a second countershock at 200 joules, resume CPR for approximately up to 30 seconds, and then reassess the rhythm. This may be repeated a third time if ventricular fibrillation persists. No more than a total of three shocks are permitted in any resuscitative event regardless of the number of EMTs at the scene. If, however, the third defibrillatory shock produced a *perfusing rhythm* and after a period of time, the patient goes back into ventricular fibrillation, *one* more defibrillatory shock may be delivered. In general, CPR should not be stopped for more than 10 seconds when assessing the cardiac rhythm. The protocol for EMT defibrillation is depicted in the schematic diagram below. The standing orders utilized in the King County, Washington, program are included in the appendix.

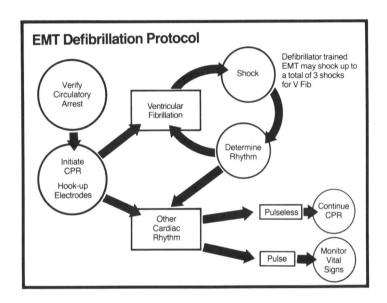

The EMT in charge of the defibrillation is also responsible for accurate documentation on the run report, for labeling paper strip and cassette recordings, and for submitting the documentation to the proper individual.

DEFIBRILLATION FOR CHILDREN

Unless it is specifically authorized by the medical director, children under the age of 12 should not be defibrillated by EMTs. Children age 12–16 should be defibrillated using 100–150 joules.

DEFIBRILLATION DURING TRANSPORT

If, while a patient is being transported, it is necessary to deliver a countershock and three shocks have not already been given, the EMT can defibrillate after proceeding in the following manner:

1. Come to a complete stop.
2. Be sure that artifact is not mistakenly identified as ventricular fibrillation. In other words, be sure that leads are properly attached and that there is no muscle movement by the patient.
3. Obtain an ECG paper strip (if available) for adequate documentation.
4. Since defibrillation poses certain hazards in a confined area with various metal objects close by, proper technique and safety guidelines must be followed when defibrillating to avoid patient and user hazard.

Arrest Prior to or After EMT Arrival

Cardiac arrest usually occurs prior to the arrival of EMTs. It is often possible to determine whether the collapse was directly witnessed by a bystander or relative, or whether the person was discovered in a state of collapse after an unknown period of time. Individuals whose arrest was directly witnessed have a better likelihood of successful resuscitation by virtue of the fact that emergency care is usually called for immediately, so that the time from collapse to delivery of emergency care is less than when an individual is down for an unknown period of time before being discovered.

There may be instances when the collapse occurs after the arrival of the Emergency Medical Technician. For example: EMTs may be called to the scene of a patient having chest pain due to a myocardial infarction. After arrival at the scene the patient may go into ventricular fibrillation. The protocol to be followed in this situation is the same as for the situation when the individual has collapsed prior to arrival. Determine lack of consciousness, lack of respiration, and lack of pulse; initiate CPR, and immediately attach the electrodes of the monitor. In situations involving collapse after arrival of the Emergency Medical Technician, it should be possible to deliver a defibrillatory shock very soon after collapse (assuming ventricular fibrillation is present). The patient has a very high likelihood of being successfully resuscitated.

Documenting the Event

Adequate documentation of the care provided in resuscitation is important for maintaining quality control of the program and for documenting successful resuscitations. Documentation should be both written and electronic. Written documentation refers to the case report filled out by the EMT following a resuscitation. This report should be sufficiently detailed so that anyone reading the report could reconstruct the events of the resuscitation. Flow charts are extremely useful in providing documentation of what occurred and in what sequence. On pages 78-79 is an example of a report completed by an EMT following a resuscitation.

Electronic documentation refers to the actual recording of the patient's cardiac rhythm. This recording should ideally be in several ways. There should be a paper strip recording of the patient's rhythm (if the machine being used allows for ECG printout). More important, however, is a cassette tape recording of the patient's heart rhythm and all voices during the resuscitation. Several defibrillators are commercially available that allow two-channel recordings of a patient's heart rhythm on one channel and voices of emergency personnel on the other channel. By means of a two-channel cassette player, the physician/director or supervisor of the program can reconstruct the resuscitation, document the specific sequence of events, and determine that the proper procedures were followed. Hence, it is important during the resuscitation to give a verbal narrative of what is occurring. For example, "This is firefighter Jones from Spanaway Fire Department at the scene of cardiac arrest. CPR is in progress. I'm beginning to hook up the electrodes; white to right shoulder, red to left ribs, green to left shoulder. Here's some quick calibrations. Beginning to assess patient's rhythm; stop CPR. Patient appears to be in ventricular fibrillation; I've gooped up the paddles. I'm charging the paddles to 175 joules. Applying paddles: stand back. One last check of rhythm; shock delivered; resume CPR."

Only with adequate documentation of the event is the EMT protected, and only with adequate documentation is the physician/director protected as well.

KING COUNTY
EMERGENCY MEDICAL SERVICES
INCIDENT REPORT

Blood Run No.						Agency Incident No.	

Mo.	Day	Yr.	07142			Agency Name	No.
0 9	1 5	8 3				UNIVERSITY F.D.	9 8

Are You First EMS Reporting Agency On Scene? 1 ☑ YES 2 ☐ NO

Incident Site & City: **4052 ESSEX AVE N.**

Responding In F.D.: **9 8**

Patient Name: **FRANK BOMAN**

SEX 1 ☑ M 2 ☐ F — Age Yr. **6 2** Mo. — Pt# **1** — AID UNIT No. **2 0** — MEDIC UNIT No. **5 2** — Geo Code **0 2**

Patient Address: **4052 ESSEX AVE N.**
City & State: **SEATTLE, WASH.**
Phone: **555-3686**

Nearest Relative Name: **EDITH BOMAN**
Relation: **WIFE**
Phone:

Private Physician Name: **ROBERT KING**
Hospital or Clinic: **UNIVERSITY HOSPITAL**
Phone:

ACTION TAKEN
1 ☐ Examine Only
2 ☑ Examine & Assist
3 ☐ No Exam (Unneeded)
4 ☐ Exam/Treatment Refused

INCIDENT CODE
Mechanism **M D**
Type **2 1 8**

SEVERITY
1 ☐ Non urgent
2 ☐ Urgent
3 ☑ Immediate Life Threat
4 ☐ Not Applicable

PROCEDURES
1 ☑ O2
2 ☐ Wound Care
3 ☐ Extrication/Rescue
4 ☐ Splinting
5 ☑ Oral Airway/Bag Mask
6 ☑ ECG Monitor
7 ☐ Esophageal Obturator
8 ☑ CPR
9 ☐ Plan A - 1
10 ☐ Plan A - 2
11 ☐ Plan B
12 ☐ Endotracheal Intubation
13 ☐ IV - Central Line
14 ☐ IV - Peripheral
15 ☑ Manual DC Shock by an EMT
16 ☐ Intracardiac Injection
17 ☐ Flutter Valve
18 ☐ Pericardiocentesis
19 ☐ Cricothyrotomy
20 ☐ Shock Trouser
21 ☐ Automatic DC Shock by an EMT
Other _____

PROCED NUMBER 12-21 ONLY	EMS NUMBER
1 5	0 0 1

ECG RHYTHM
1 ☐ Sinus
2 ☐ V Fib
3 ☐ V Tach
4 ☐ Asystole
5 ☐ Idioventricular
6 ☐ Other
7 ☐ Unknown

DR. CONTACTED 1 ☑ YES 2 ☐ NO
Name of Doctor and Hospital Contacted:
1. **MEDIC #512 DR. LERCH** 2. _____
   UNIVERSITY HOSPITAL

CPR

CPR INITIATED BY
1 ☑ Fire Department
2 ☑ Paramedic
3 ☐ Ambulance
4 ☐ MD/RN
5 ☐ Citizen with Dispatcher Assistance
6 ☐ Citizen without Dispatcher Assistance

NAME OF CITIZEN INITIATING CPR
JANET HELMS
Phone **555-3771**
WAS CITIZEN PREVIOUSLY TRAINED?
1 ☐ Yes 2 ☐ No 3 ☐ Unknown

LOCATION OF CARDIAC ARREST:
1 ☑ Home
2 ☐ Residence other than home
3 ☐ Work
4 ☐ Public place
5 ☐ Nursing home
6 ☐ Other

WAS CARDIAC ARREST WITNESSED?
1 ☑ Yes 2 ☐ No
3 ☐ Unknown
WAS DISPATCHER-ASSISTED CPR OFFERED?
1 ☑ Yes 2 ☐ No
3 ☐ Unknown

ESTIMATED TIME FROM COLLAPSE TO: (Min.)
Agency Call **0 1**
Initiation Of CPR **0 4**
Definitive Care **1 0**

OUTCOME
1 ☐ Expired At Scene/ER
2 ☑ Admit To ICU/CCU
3 ☐ Unknown

Time Of Call (24 Hr.)	Response Time (Min.)		Out Of Service Time (Min.)		Source Of Alarm:	Responding From Quarters?	Transported To:	
1 9 4 1	AID	0 4	AID		1 ☑ Citizen	1 ☑ Yes	UNIV. HOSP.	2 9
					2 ☐ Police		Transported By:	
					3 ☐ MD/RN	1 ☐ No	MEDIC 512	5 2
					4 ☐ F.D.			
	MEDIC	1 0	MEDIC		5 ☐ Ambulance		Ambulance Response Time (Min.)	
					6 ☐ Other			

FOR AGENCY USE:

PERSONNEL AID
1 JOHN LUPTON, EMT-D
2 KATHY PETERSON
3 JOE RAMIREZ

PARAMEDIC
1
2
3

EMS NUMBER

SIGNATURE OF PERSON COMPLETING REPORT
John Lupton

VITAL SIGNS	POSITION	BLOOD PRESSURE	PULSE RATE	RESPIRATORY RATE	CONSCIOUSNESS	PUPILS
	← →	0 /	0	0 / Min. Est. Air Exchange	☐ Alert	☐ • Conjugate ☐ Reactive ☑ Unreactive
	↑ ↓	/		☐ Normal	☐ Semi-Conscious	☑ Dilated
TIME	↕	/		☐ Increased ☐ Decreased	☑ Comatose	☐ Dysconjugate ☐ Mid ☐ Constricted

FLOW CHART	TIME →	1946	1959	2001	2002									
	Blood Pressure	0	144/92	140/94	126/94									
	Pulse Rate	0	110	120	120									
	Respiratory Rate	0	8/M	8/M	8/M									
	Consciousness	COM	COM	COM	COM									
	Pupils	F&D	M≈R	M≈R	M≈R									
	Rhythm (ECG)	VF	3° BLK	3° BLK	—									
	Morphine													
	Oxygen	11 LT	11 LT	11 LT	11 LT									
	DC Shock (200 JOULES)	YES												

Medications Taken By Patient At Home

Narrative (Subjective, Objective, Assessment, Plan)

S. A 62 YR OLD ♂ CARDIAC ARREST. PTS WIFE STATED THAT HER HUSBAND HAD BEEN HAVING SOME CHEST PAIN EARLIER TODAY AND HAD JUST STOPPED BREATHING SHORTLY BEFORE OUR ARRIVAL. SHE ALSO STATED THAT PT. HAD JUST COME OUT OF THE HOSPITAL LAST FRIDAY. PMH$_x$: MEDICAL – ANGINA, CHF – MEDS: UNKNOWN

O. UPON ARRIVAL PT. WAS SUPINE ON LIVING ROOM FLOOR – UNCONSCIOUS, UNRESPONSIVE, NO PULSE, NO RESP., AND CYANOTIC IN COLOR, NO LIFE SIGNS. C.P.R. WAS NOT IN PROGRESS UPON ARRIVAL BUT WAS ATTEMPTED BY WIFE PRIOR TO OUR ARRIVAL. HEENT – PUP FIX AND DILATED, NECK VEINS DISTENT, PT CYANOTIC, ECG – VENT-FIB

ASS. CARDIAC ARR.

PLAN – C.P.R. INITIATED UPON ARRIVAL - HEART MONITOR HOOK-UP – I COUNTERSHOCK ADMIN. PRIOR TO MEDIC 512 ARRIVAL – STRIP IS ATTACHED – BAG MASK WITH 100% O$_2$ @ 11 LITERS. BASIC LIFE SUPPORT ADMIN. APPROX 6 MIN BEFORE PT LIFE SIGNS CAME BACK. MEDIC 512 ALSO ADMIN I.V. & LIDOCAINE, ATROPINE @ APPROX 1956 HOURS TRANS TO U.H. VIA MEDIC 512 WITH REQUIRED BAG MASK ASSIST ONLY.

FORM 911 1/83

Chapter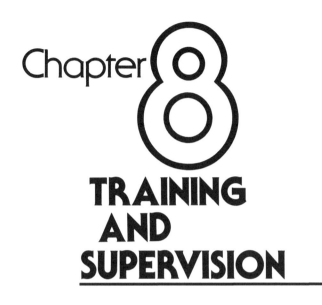

TRAINING AND SUPERVISION

Training Requirements

Training requirements for an EMT Defibrillation Program will vary from community to community depending upon experience of EMTs, volume of calls, local facilities, and many other factors unique to each community. The physician/director, since he or she is responsible for the medical performance of defibrillation-trained EMTs, must decide how much training is required.

The appendix contains the instructors' guide for EMT Defibrillation Courses in Washington State. A typical course requires 10 hours (not including testing time) and consists of four sessions. The first session is a CPR review. The second is a three-hour lecture discussing the material contained in this textbook. The third is a four-hour practical session learning about the operation of a defibrillator, practicing on an Arrhythmia Anne, and interpreting various cardiac rhythms. The last session consists of a practical and written test.

An optional part of the training program can be an experience defibrillating an anesthetized dog. Depending upon the availability of an animal laboratory and means to fund such a session, the experience of delivering a DC shock to a living creature can boost confidence and better prepare the EMT for rapid decision-making.

CONTINUING EDUCATION REQUIREMENTS

Maintaining the skill of EMT defibrillation requires continued practice and review. Each program must decide upon its own continuing education resources and requirements. Generally, we recommend at least four continuing education classes per year. These classes should be 1–2 hours in length and should include practice in simulated cardiac arrest using Arrhythmia Anne as well as a review of resuscitations that have occurred in the previous months. Review of the standing orders and periodic reviews of basic cardiac rhythms should also be a part of such classes.

EMT defibrillation requires a committment to continued learning. The ability to constructively review the performance of an EMT is an important part of the program.

Physician Supervision

An EMT Defibrillation Program, in order to operate safely, must have a physician Medical Director. EMT defibrillation, while potentially lifesaving, is also potentially dangerous. If used inappropriately by untrained or undertrained individuals, and if improper supervision exists, harm may result.

RESPONSIBILITIES OF THE MEDICAL DIRECTOR

The Medical Director is ultimately responsible for all aspects of the program. It is her/his job to maintain close medical supervision of the program and to ensure high skill and performance levels in EMTs trained to defibrillate. The responsibilities of the Medical Director include:

1. Participation in the training program, through either direct teaching or supervision of the training.
2. Permission for EMTs to participate in the program.
3. Written authorization of standing orders.
4. Supervision of a continuing education program.
5. Review and documentation of each resuscitation in which EMT defibrillation care is delivered.
6. Establishment and maintenance of individual case records.
7. Rescinding of permission for EMTs to participate for any of the following reasons:
    a. Nonprofessional behavior or attitude.
    b. Nonadherence to standing orders.
    c. Nonparticipation in continuing education classes.
    d. Failure to demonstrate high performance.

The responsibilities of the Medical Director cannot be taken lightly; close and continuous supervision is required.

EMT Defibrillation in Rural Communities

Though smaller communities (with populations of 30,000 and fewer) may potentially have the most to gain from the implementation of EMT defibrillation (EMT-D) level services, we would like to urge special caution upon EMTs and Directors and Medical Directors of ambulance services in such communities. EMT-D care can be provided safely and effectively by medium and high volume services located in suburban and urban settings. However, for rural communities with a low volume of cardiac arrests, special problems must be addressed. A controlled study has assessed the impact of EMT defibrillation on rural emergency cardiac care in Iowa and has also helped to identify problems unique to the rural environment.

The major problem in rural programs is the low frequency of skill usage by the EMT. In Iowa, for example, a typical small town ambulance service is staffed by 18–20 volunteer EMTs who work full-time at other occupations, usually unrelated to medical care. The ambulance service responds, on the average, to 3–5 out-of-hospital cardiac arrests per year. Any given EMT, then, will participate in the resuscitation of no more than one or two patients per year, and perhaps even fewer. Ensuring that *all* EMTs will be able to perform the skills of assessment and defibrillation quickly, accurately, and safely when and if their time comes is a major concern. Experience in rural Iowa has identified two major deficiencies resulting from infrequent skill use: (1) fear and lack of confidence, which contribute to (2) deterioration in skill speed. Provider fear translates into a hesitation to use the machine, but appears to be rooted in a fear of misinterpreting a rhythm and delivering a shock inappropriately, and/or a fear of operating the equipment incorrectly. Instances have been documented where up to six minutes have elapsed between the initial recognition of ventricular fibrillation and the delivery of the first shock. Patients who were subjected to such delays in treatment, of course, did not survive.

The best solution to deal with infrequent skill utilization is regular periodic training sessions. The use of a standardized simulated cardiac arrest exercise in which all EMT-Ds are required to perform at least quarterly can prevent skill degradation. The format of the simulation should include potential machine malfunctions, artifactual rhythms, and other stumbling blocks that have been identified as potentially resulting in inappropriate or delayed patient treatment. The use of the simulations is cumbersome, time-consuming, difficult to enforce and monitor, and not without cost; but it can result in improved speed and efficiency. We feel that such a system is absolutely necessary in order to maintain an effective low-volume EMT-D level ambulance service.

It is also essential that all actual cardiac arrest calls be reviewed within a very few days of their occurrence by a designated qualified individual. The only way we know of to adequately review these calls is through the use of a cassette tape voice/ECG recorder equipped heart monitor. The tapes must be reviewed promptly in order to provide immediate feedback, positive as well as negative, to the EMTs. The tape reviewer ideally might be the ambulance service Medical Director, though often the physician is too busy to take on this responsibility. If that is the case, the individual designated for the task must, at a minimum, be qualified in ACLS, and be in a position of authority with respect to the ambulance service. It would be best if this individual had considerable experience with the management of out-of-hospital cardiac arrest so that individual runs could be analyzed on the basis of experience. Because of the limited number of cardiac arrest calls in any given rural community we believe that a centralized approach to both run reviews and practice simulation reviews works very well. For example, the activities of every EMT-D service in Iowa are overseen by a single panel of reviewers who report back to the individual Medical Directors and EMTs. This system has several advantages. (1) A resuscitation attempt can be evaluated in the context of 40–50 other resuscitations per year instead of one or two. (2) Runs are reviewed promptly using standard criteria, and written reports are generated for the record. (3) Centralized data collection is easily accomplished, allowing ongoing evaluation of the program as a whole as well as for individual services.

It is our belief that EMT defibrillation has the potential to significantly improve rural emergency care. Such services must, however, be developed and maintained with great care and with a high concern for safety and effectiveness.

Appendix 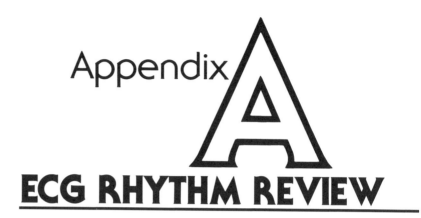 A

ECG RHYTHM REVIEW

Normal Sinus Rhythm

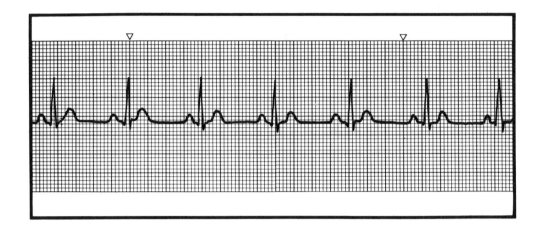

CHARACTERISTICS
1. **QRS Complexes:**
   a. Narrow and tight.
   b. Normal conduction of < 0.12 seconds.
   c. Uniform in shape.
   d. Regular.
2. **P Waves:**
   a. There is a P wave for every QRS.
   b. Slight variation in shape likely to be caused by patient or cable movement.
   c. PR interval is normal at < 0.20 seconds.
   d. Rate is constant.
3. **Rate:**
   a. Atrial: 70 per minute.
   b. Ventricular: 70 per minute.

SIGNIFICANCE
Normal sinus rhythm indicates that the origin of impulse is from the SA node. Conduction of that impulse proceeds in sequence through the atrium to the AV node, down the bundle of His and the bundle branches, and out to the ventricular muscle cells by way of the Purkinje fibers. This is a healthy rhythm and indicates normal function throughout the electrical system.

ADDITIONAL EXAMPLES

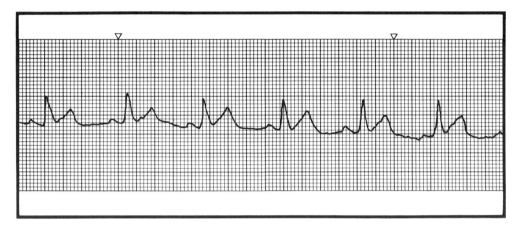

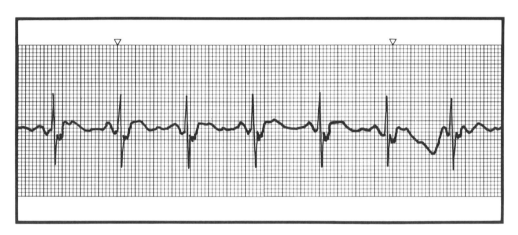

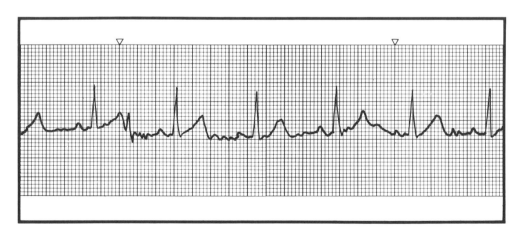

Sinus Arrhythmia

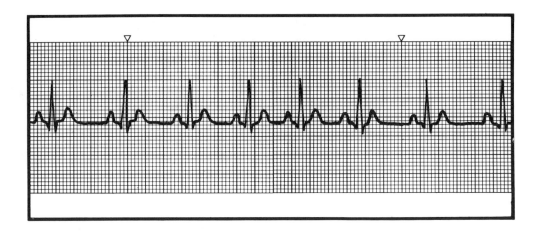

CHARACTERISTICS
1. **QRS Complexes:**
   a. Narrow and tight.
   b. Normal conduction: < 0.12 seconds.
   c. The intervals between QRS complexes vary.
2. **P Waves:**
   a. Before each QRS complex.
   b. Uniform in appearance.
   c. PR interval normal: < 0.2 seconds.
3. **Rate:**
   a. Atrial: 75 per minute.
   b. Ventricular: 75 per minute.

SIGNIFICANCE
The slight beat-to-beat irregularity is related to changes brought about by respirations. This rhythm is commonly found in healthy children or athletic adults.

INTERVENTION
1. Assess the patient and obtain history.
2. Treat specific complaint or injuries.
3. Administer oxygen only if indicated.

ADDITIONAL EXAMPLE

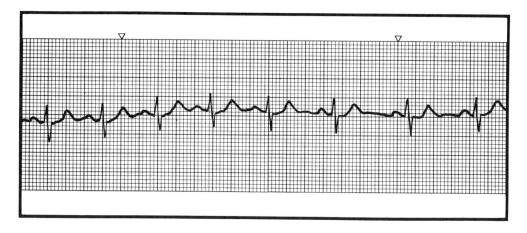

Sinus Tachycardia

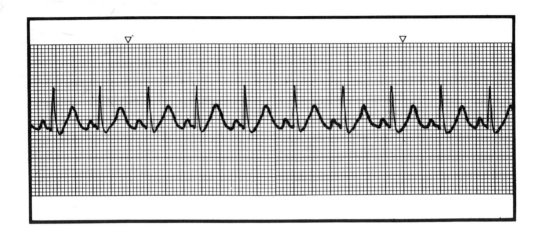

CHARACTERISTICS
1. **QRS Complexes:**
   a. Narrow and tight.
   b. Uniform in shape.
   c. Conduction normal at < 0.12 seconds.
   d. Rhythm regular.
2. **P Waves:**
   a. P wave for every QRS complex.
   b. Uniform in shape.
   c. PR interval normal at < 0.2 seconds.
   d. Regular.
3. **Rate:**
   a. Atrial: 105 per minute.
   b. Ventricular: 105 per minute.

SIGNIFICANCE

Sinus tachycardia represents an accelerated discharge of electrical impulses from the SA node. An increased heart rate can occur as a natural response to normal physiological conditions or to illness and injury. Fear, anxiety, pain, and physical exercise can induce tachycardia as can certain stimulants, such as caffeine and nicotine. In certain pathological conditions—such as shock, congestive heart failure, and acute myocardial infarction—in which there is a decrease in the cardiac output or blood pressure, the body will attempt to compensate by increasing the heart rate.

Because sinus tachycardia is a normal response to an underlying condition, treatment is directed at identifying and eliminating the causative agent.

INTERVENTION

1. Identify underlying cause and treat accordingly.
2. Administer oxygen.
3. Continue cardiac monitoring; watch for changes in rate or rhythm.

ADDITIONAL EXAMPLES

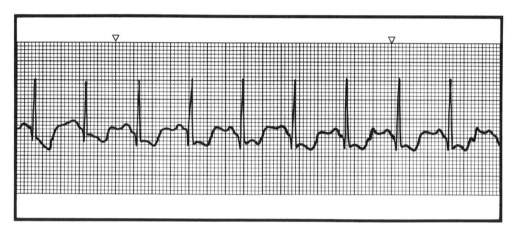

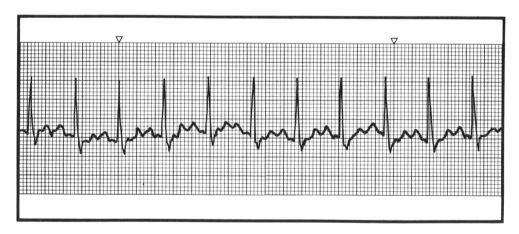

Supraventricular Tachycardia

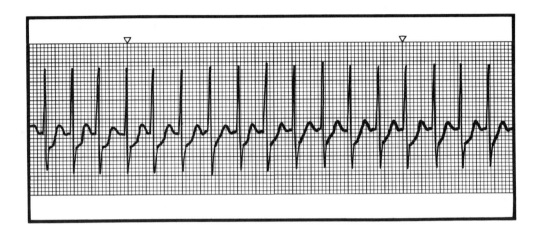

CHARACTERISTICS

Supraventricular tachycardia (SVT) is a generalized term used to identify any tachycardia originating above the ventricles in which the atrial mechanism is unclear. The P wave may be hidden because the ventricular rate is so rapid, making it difficult to determine whether the impulse started in the SA node, the atria, or the AV junction.

Since the pacing site in SVT is above the ventricles, the QRS complex will generally be normal in shape and conduction. This is in comparison to an impulse originating in the ventricles—outside the normal conduction pathway—in which the QRS complex is wide and bizarre-looking.

Distinguishing between ventricular tachycardia (VT) and supraventricular tachycardia (SVT) can usually be done quickly on the basis of the QRS complex. If the QRS complex is narrow and tight, the impulse originates above the ventricles; if the QRS complex is wide and bizarre, the impulse originates in the ventricles.

SIGNIFICANCE

The significance with any tachycardia is in the patient's ability to tolerate a rapid heart rate. If the heart rate is too fast, the ventricles do not have time to fill with enough blood. Thus there is a reduction in the amount of blood pumped with each heart beat. The patient might experience lightheadedness, dizziness, hypotension, angina, or even loss of consciousness. Treatment of the patient is dictated by his/her symptoms.

INTERVENTION
1. Assess patient's vital signs and physical condition.
2. Provide basic life support as indicated.
3. Administer oxygen, position comfortably, and continue to monitor vital signs while awaiting paramedics.

ADDITIONAL EXAMPLES

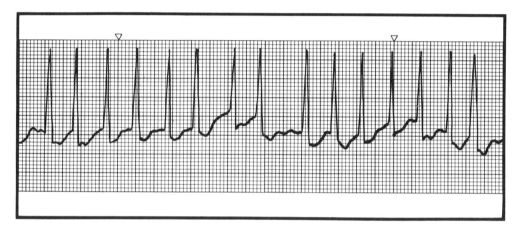

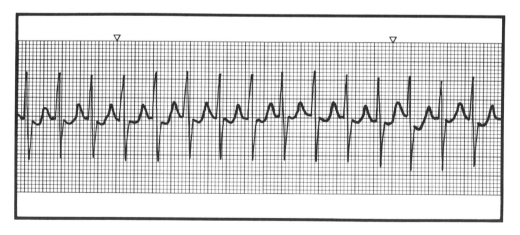

Sinus Bradycardia

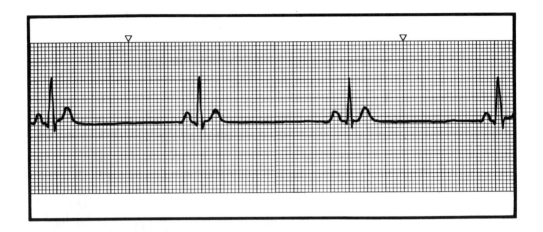

CHARACTERISTICS
1. **QRS Complexes:**
   a. Narrow and tight.
   b. Uniform in shape.
   c. Normal conduction: <0.12 seconds.
   d. Rhythm regular.
2. **P Waves:**
   a. Precede each QRS complex.
   b. Each P wave is uniform.
   c. PR interval is constant and normal at <0.20 seconds.
3. **Rate:**
   a. Atrial: 37 per minute.
   b. Ventricular: 37 per minute.

SIGNIFICANCE
The formation and transmission of impulses from the SA node is slowed to a rate less than 60 beats per minute. In some instances, this may be a normal condition—particularly among athletic individuals whose resting heart rate may be as low as 45.

In other cases, sinus bradycardia may signify more serious conditions. Severe hypoxia, or lack of oxygen, can slow the heart rate. Certain drugs, such as digitalis or antiarrhythmics, can cause bradycardia. Elderly patients may be bradycardic as a result of degenerative heart disease.

Depending on the patient's underlying condition, sinus bradycardia may cause lightheadedness and fainting. Severe bradycardia, generally less than 40, can result in a significant reduction in blood flow to the brain and vital organs, causing unconsciousness and possibly cardiac arrest.

INTERVENTION
1. If patient is unconscious, determine need for CPR.
2. If patient is conscious, administer oxygen, conduct primary assessment with vital signs.
3. Continue to monitor for possible deterioration while awaiting paramedic arrival.

ADDITIONAL EXAMPLES

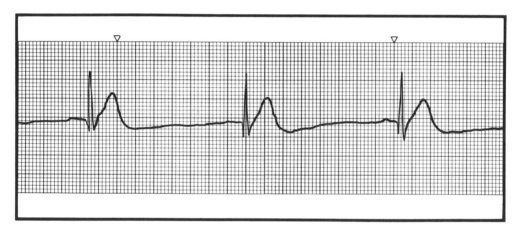

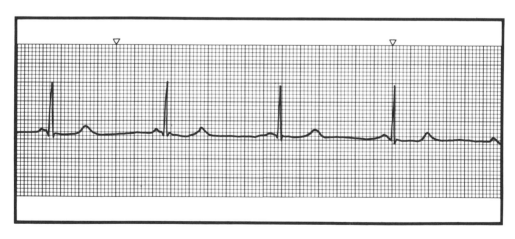

Atrial Flutter

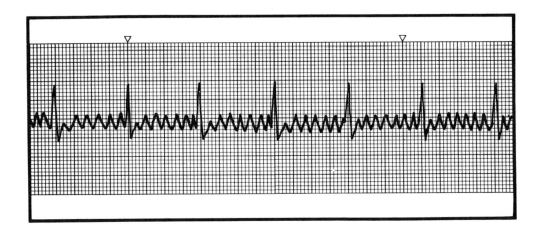

CHARACTERISTICS
1. **QRS Complexes:**
   a. Narrow and tight.
   b. Conduction normal: < 0.12 seconds.
   c. Uniform in shape.
   d. Rhythm slightly irregular.
2. **P Waves:**
   a. In atrial flutter, the P waves are referred to as *flutter waves,* of which there are several interspersed between QRS complexes.
   b. The flutter waves march out regularly, several being hidden within the QRS and T wave.
   c. The flutter waves resemble a sawtooth pattern.
3. **Rate:**
   a. Atrial: 50 per minute.
   b. Ventricular: 40 per minute.

SIGNIFICANCE
In atrial flutter, the atria are stimulated by a focus outside the SA node, causing the atrium to contract rapidly. The atrial rate is generally between 250 to 350 beats per minute. Obviously, not all the atrial beats are conducted to the ventricles, since the ventricular rate varies from the atrial rate.

This rhythm is rarely seen in people with healthy hearts. It can occur in patients with heart disease, acute myocardial infarction, hypoxia, lung disease, and pulmonary embolism.

The ability of the patient to tolerate this rhythm is dependent upon his/her underlying condition and the rate at which the ventricles respond. The patient may become compromised if the ventricular rate is either too slow or too fast.

INTERVENTION
1. Assess level of consciousness and vital signs.
2. Administer oxygen.
3. Provide basic life support as indicated.
4. Continue to monitor while awaiting paramedic arrival.

ADDITIONAL EXAMPLES

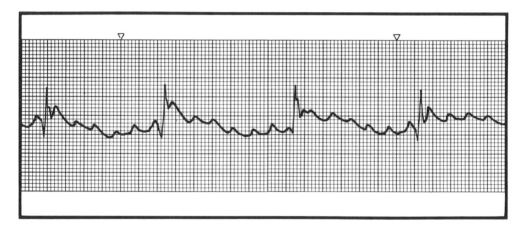

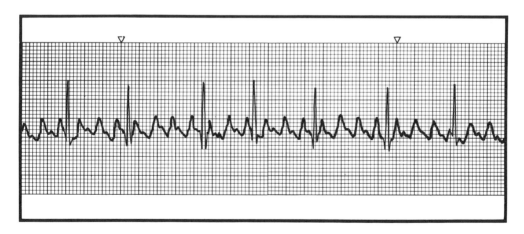

Atrial Fibrillation

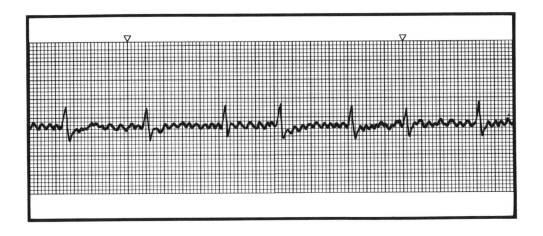

CHARACTERISTICS
1. **QRS Complexes:**
   a. Narrow.
   b. Uniform in shape.
   c. Conduction is < 0.12 seconds.
   d. Rhythm is irregularly irregular.
2. **P Waves:**
   a. No regular, uniform P waves appear.
   b. Baseline is rippling.
3. **Ventricular Rate:** Approximately 80.

SIGNIFICANCE
With atrial fibrillation, the cells within the atria are firing chaotically and independently. There is no coordinated, rhythmic contraction of the atria. Electrical impulses from the atria are conducted through the AV node to the ventricles irregularly. Conduction through the ventricles is normal.

Atrial fibrillation is seen most often with patients in congestive heart failure owing to the overstretching of the atrium. The rhythm may or may not be tolerated, depending upon the rate of ventricular response and the patient's underlying disease.

INTERVENTION
1. Assess level of consciousness and vital signs.
2. Administer oxygen.
3. Determine severity of condition for possible paramedic intervention.
4. Continue to monitor.

ADDITIONAL EXAMPLES

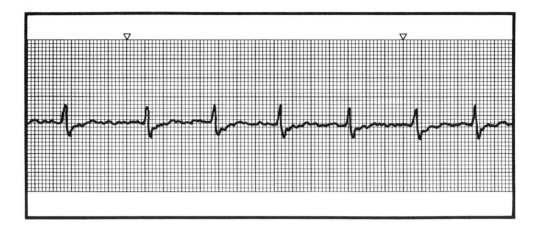

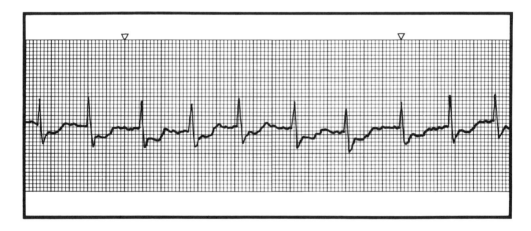

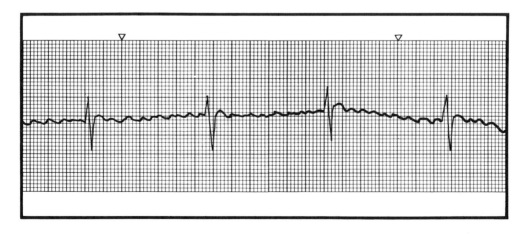

Nodal Rhythm

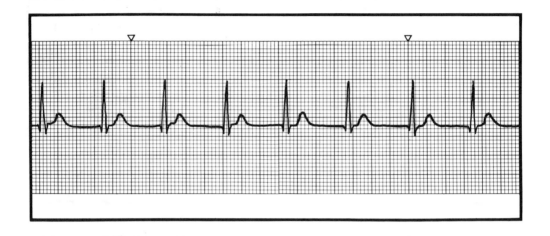

CHARACTERISTICS
1. **QRS Complexes:**
   a. Narrow and tight.
   b. Normal conduction: <0.12 seconds.
   c. Consistent and uniform.
   d. Regular.
2. **P Waves:** Absent.
3. **Rate:** Ventricular rate is 100 per minute.

SIGNIFICANCE
Nodal rhythm occurs when the SA node fails to function. Other parts of the conduction system, as, in this case, the AV junction, can assume the role of pacemaker in initiating an electrical impulse and can produce a rhythm. This is known as *automaticity.*

This rhythm has a normal-appearing QRS complex and T wave, but there is no recognizable P wave. This implies that the impulse originated outside the atrium but above the bundle of His.

A nodal rhythm may occur in the setting of digitalis toxicity, acute myocardial infarction, and hypoxia. The rate may become excessively slow, requiring oxygen and specific medications.

INTERVENTION
1. Determine level of responsiveness.
2. Assess adequacy of airway and respirations.
3. Verify presence or absence of pulse.
4. Provide basic life support as indicated.
5. If patient is conscious, administer oxygen.
6. Monitor vital signs. Watch for possible deterioration.

ADDITIONAL EXAMPLES

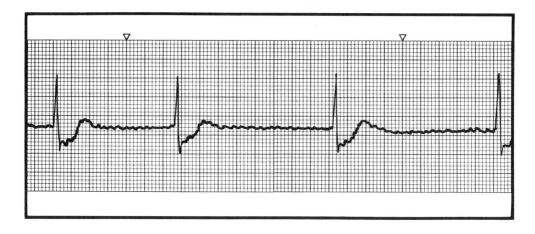

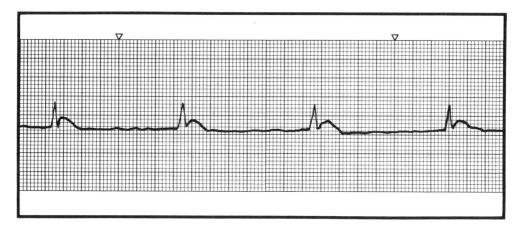

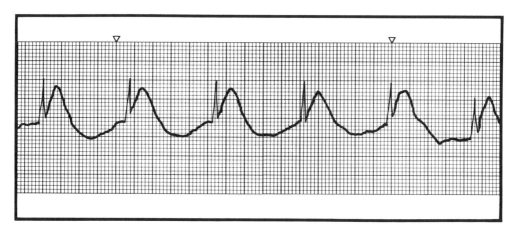

First-Degree Heart Block *Slowing through the node*

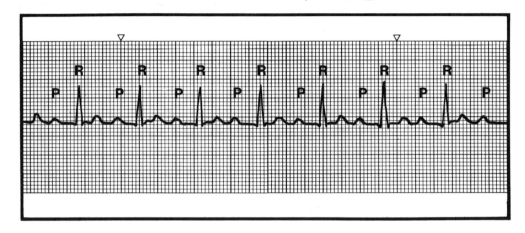

CHARACTERISTICS
1. **QRS Complexes:**
   a. Narrow and tight.
   b. Uniform.
   c. Conduction: <0.12 seconds.
   d. Regular rhythm.
2. **P Waves:**
   a. P wave precedes each QRS complex.
   b. P waves are uniform.
   c. PR interval is constant, but abnormally prolonged at 0.28 seconds (normal: <0.20 seconds).
3. **Rate:** 75 per minute.

SIGNIFICANCE

First-degree heart block (1°HB) occurs when there is delayed conduction of an impulse through the AV node. This can be determined by the presence of a prolonged PR interval that is greater than 0.20 seconds.

Conditions causing first-degree heart block can also cause second- and third-degree heart block. Ischemic heart disease, acute myocardial infarction, and specific drugs can cause AV heart block. If 1°HB is associated with severe bradycardia, the patient might be hypotensive and unconscious.

INTERVENTION
1. Provide basic life support as needed.
2. If conscious, administer oxygen and conduct vital workup.
3. Continue to monitor while awaiting paramedic arrival.

ADDITIONAL EXAMPLES

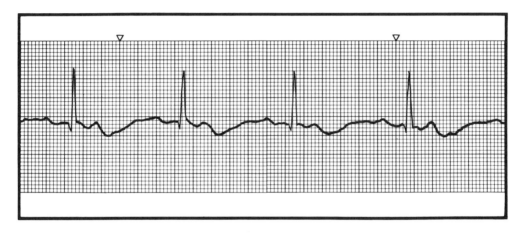

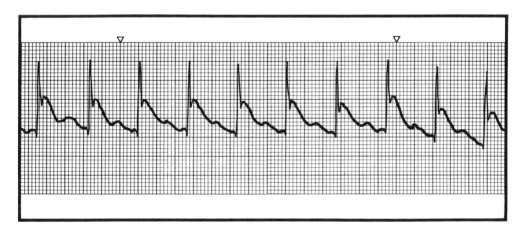

Second-Degree Heart Block, Mobitz Type I (Wenckebach)

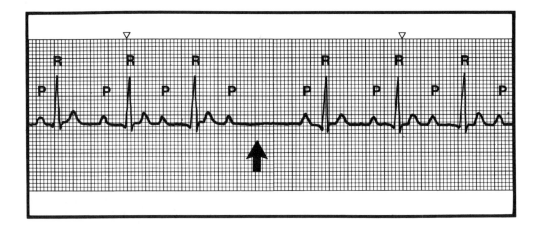

CHARACTERISTICS
1. **QRS Complexes:**
   a. Narrow and tight.
   b. Uniform in shape.
   c. Normal conduction: <0.12 seconds.
   d. Rhythm irregular.
2. **P Waves:**
   a. P waves are present and uniform in shape.
   b. PR interval progressively lengthens until a QRS beat is dropped (indicated by ↑).
3. **Rate:**
   a. Atrial: 100 per minute.
   b. Ventricular: 60 per minute.

SIGNIFICANCE
Mobitz type I, or Wenckebach, is a form of second-degree heart block in which conduction of the sinus impulse is progressively delayed through the AV node until no conduction occurs. This is seen when a P wave is followed by a long pause without a QRS complex. The blocked beat allows the AV node to recover and the whole cycle repeats itself.

This type of heart block is considered less serious than Mobitz type II, and often is temporary. Unless the ventricular rate is slow, the patient is usually without symptoms.

Causes of Mobitz type I heart block include ischemic heart

disease, acute myocardial infarction, and digitalis toxicity. Depending on the underlying cause, the patient may develop complete heart block. Close monitoring is necessary to observe any change in condition.

INTERVENTION
1. Administer oxygen.
2. Continue to monitor, recording vital signs, while awaiting paramedics.

ADDITIONAL EXAMPLES

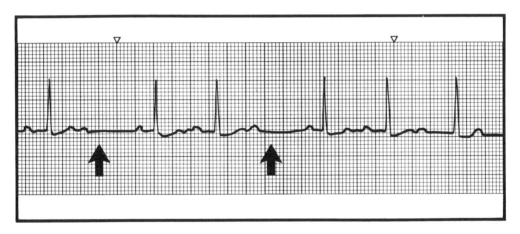

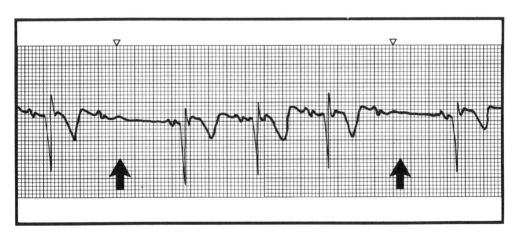

Second-Degree Heart Block, Mobitz Type II

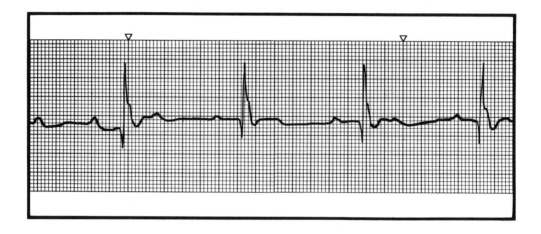

CHARACTERISTICS
1. **QRS Complexes:**
   a. Uniform in shape.
   b. Occur regularly.
   c. Conduction is normal: < 0.12 seconds.
2. **P Waves:**
   a. Two P waves for each QRS complex.
   b. Occur regularly.
   c. PR interval constant, but prolonged (greater than 0.20 seconds).
3. **Rate:**
   a. Atrial: 100 per minute.
   b. Ventricular: 40 per minute.

SIGNIFICANCE
Mobitz type II heart block is characterized by a series of non-conducted P waves followed by a P wave that is conducted. The interval at which a P wave is actually conducted through the AV node may vary. In the above example, the ratio of nonconducted to conducted impulses is 2:1. In other examples, the ratio may be 3:1 or 4:1.

This type of block represents a more serious impairment of the conduction system. It often occurs as a result of acute myocardial infarction, and commonly progresses to complete heart block.

INTERVENTION
1. Administer oxygen.
2. Provide basic life support as needed.
3. Continue to monitor closely for signs of deterioration until paramedics arrive.

ADDITIONAL EXAMPLES

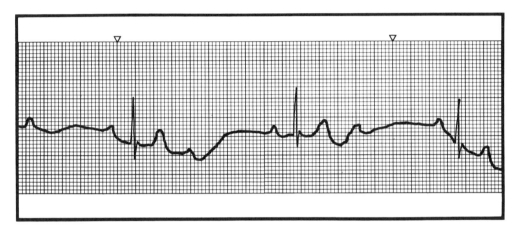

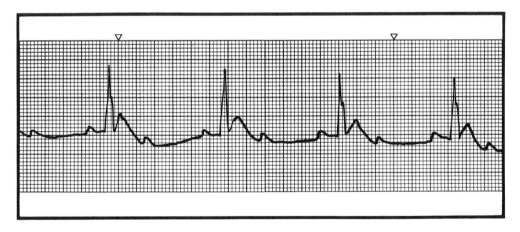

Third-Degree Heart Block

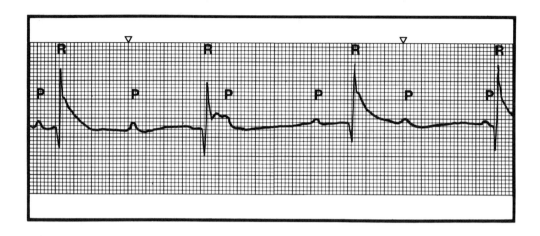

CHARACTERISTICS
1. **QRS Complexes:**
   a. May be narrow and tight or wide and bizarre.
   b. Conduction may be normal (<0.12 seconds) or abnormally prolonged.
   c. Complexes may be uniform or varying in appearance.
   d. Rhythm may be regular or very irregular.
2. **P Waves:**
   a. Present and occur at a regular interval.
   b. Do not have fixed, constant relationship to the QRS complex.
   c. PR interval abnormally prolonged and changing.
3. **Rate:**
   a. Atrial: 75 per minute.
   b. Ventricular: 40 per minute.

SIGNIFICANCE

Heart block occurs when there is impaired conduction of impulses through the AV node. Third-degree heart block is the most serious and extreme form.

Heart block may be transient and incomplete, allowing some impulses to be conducted from the atria through the AV junction to the ventricles, as with first- or second-degree heart block. With complete or third-degree block, there is no transmission of impulses from the atria to the ventricles. The atria and ventricles are paced independently of one another.

Third-degree heart block occurs more commonly in older patients with chronic degenerative changes in their conduction system. It can also occur with digitalis toxicity or with acute myocardial infarction.

INTERVENTION
1. Determine level of consciousness and responsiveness.
2. Assess adequacy of airway and respirations.
3. Verify presence or absence of pulse.
4. Provide basic life support if indicated.
5. If patient is conscious, administer oxygen.
6. Because of the seriousness of this rhythm, request paramedics or immediately transport to emergency room facility.

ADDITIONAL EXAMPLES

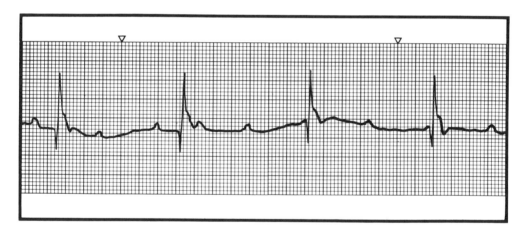

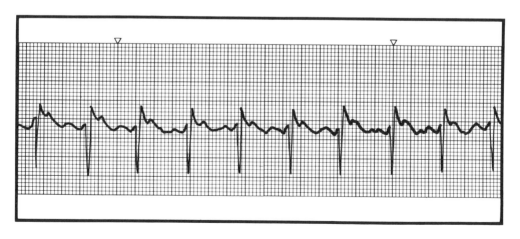

Premature Ventricular Contractions: Unifocal

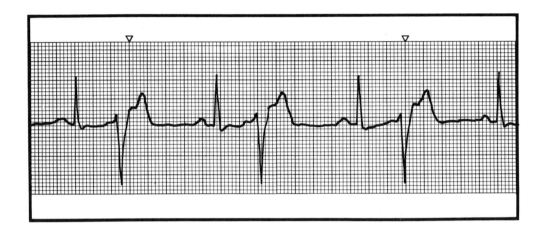

CHARACTERISTICS
1. **QRS Complexes:**
   a. Dominant QRS complexes narrow and tight.
      (1) Conduction time normal at <0.12 seconds.
   b. Premature QRS complexes wide and bizarre.
      (1) Conduction time >0.12 seconds (0.14 seconds in this example).
      (2) Uniform in shape, indicating that they occurred from the same site: unifocal.
2. **P Waves:**
   a. Precede every *normal* QRS.
   b. Uniform in shape.
   c. PR interval normal at <0.20 seconds.
   d. Occur at a constant rate, and are hidden in the premature beats.
3. **Rate:** 90 per minute.

SIGNIFICANCE
A premature ventricular contraction is the result of an electrical impulse being discharged somewhere within the ventricles but outside the normal conduction pathway, stimulating the ventricles to contract early. Associated with chest pain or cardiac disease, PVCs may indicate a serious condition. In patients experiencing chest pain, the presence of PVCs can signify ischemia or severe myocardial injury. The patient is very likely to suddenly develop ventricular tachycardia or to suffer sudden death.

INTERVENTION
1. Assess for possible myocardial infarction.
2. Administer oxygen.
3. Follow protocol for treating MI.
4. Monitor rhythm closely for further deterioration.

ADDITIONAL EXAMPLES

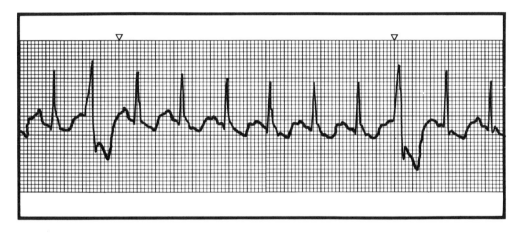

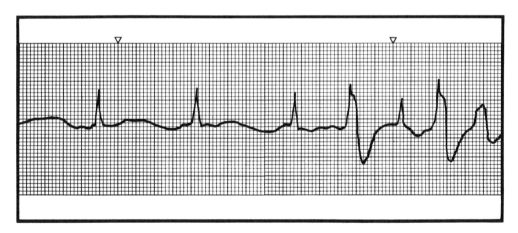

Ventricular Tachycardia

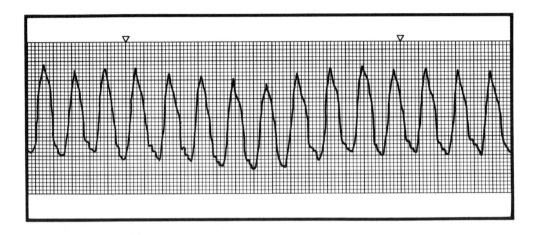

CHARACTERISTICS
1. **QRS Complexes:**
   a. Wide and bizarre.
   b. Uniform in shape with slight variation.
   c. Prolonged conduction at > 0.12 seconds.
   d. Rhythm regular.
2. **P Waves:** Absent.
3. **Rate:** Ventricular rate is 150.

SIGNIFICANCE
Ventricular tachycardia is a life-threatening arrhythmia. The rapid rate diminishes adequate cardiac output, causing severe hypotension. The patient may be conscious with a decreased blood pressure, or unconscious and pulseless. This rhythm generally deteriorates into ventricular fibrillation.

Heart disease, angina, myocardial infarction, electrolyte imbalances, hypoxia, and drugs can cause ventricular tachycardia. Premature ventricular contractions, often associated with acute myocardial infarction, can also trigger ventricular tachycardia

INTERVENTION
1. Verify presence or absence of cardiopulmonary arrest.
2. Provide basic life support as indicated.
3. If patient is conscious, administer oxygen.
4. Prepare for defibrillation in case rhythm deteriorates to ventricular fibrillation.

ADDITIONAL EXAMPLES

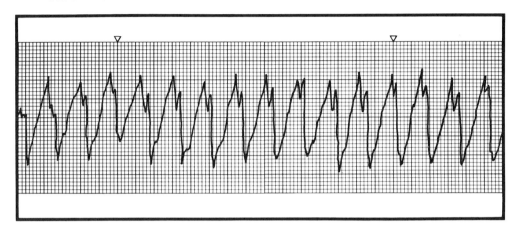

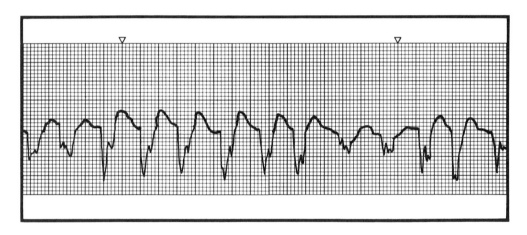

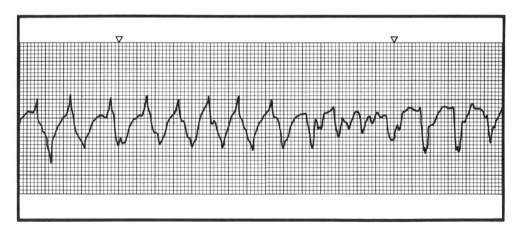

Ventricular Flutter

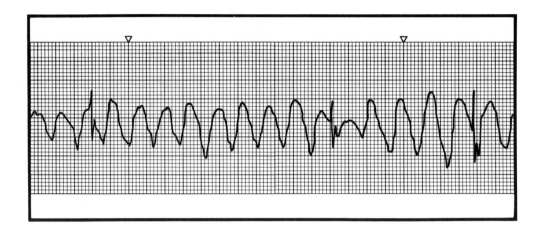

CHARACTERISTICS
1. **QRS Complexes:**
   a. Varied and bizarre.
   b. Varied in amplitude and shape.
   c. Conduction abnormally long (0.28 seconds in this example.)
   d. Rhythm slightly irregular.
2. **P Waves:** Absent.
3. **Rate:** Ventricular rate is 150 per minute.

SIGNIFICANCE
Ventricular flutter is a worsening progression of ventricular tachycardia. This rhythm heralds the onset of ventricular fibrillation as the myocardium becomes more ischemic. With prolonged lack of oxygen, the electrical conduction becomes impaired, the QRS complexes begin to dampen, and the rhythm becomes irregular as it approaches the chaotic disorder of ventricular fibrillation.

INTERVENTION
1. With the loss of pulse and blood pressure, begin CPR.
2. Prepare to defibrillate as the rhythm deteriorates to ventricular fibrillation.

ADDITIONAL EXAMPLES

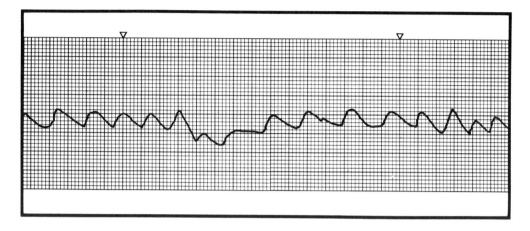

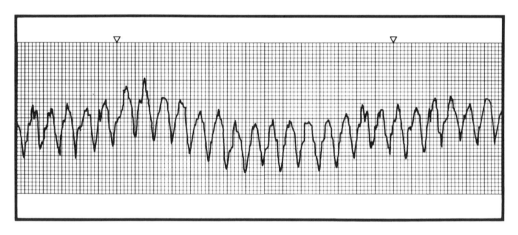

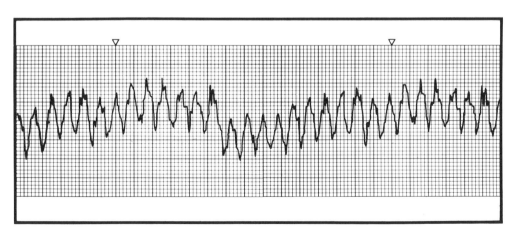

Ventricular Fibrillation

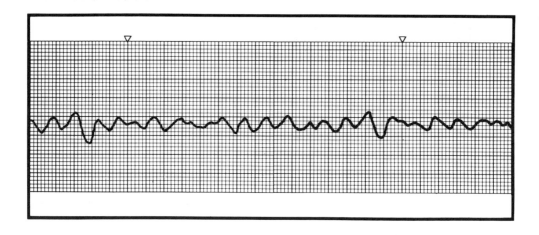

CHARACTERISTICS
1. **QRS Complexes:**
   a. Absence of normal-looking complexes.
   b. Baseline wavy, chaotic, and inconsistent.
   c. Rhythm irregular.
2. **P Waves:** Absent.
3. **Rate:** Indeterminate.

SIGNIFICANCE
Sudden death and cardiac arrest immediately follow the onset of ventricular fibrillation. The patient will be unconscious, unresponsive, without respirations and pulse.

The fibrillatory waves indicate the absence of any coordinated, rhythmic contraction of the heart. The heart, if visualized, would be quivering or twitching, unable to pump blood.

The pattern of waves often changes from coarse to fine fibrillation. The only definite treatment for ventricular fibrillation is immediate defibrillation.

This rhythm may occur in association with heart disease of any type. It may be preceded by warning arrhythmias, such as PVCs or ventricular tachycardia, or it may occur spontaneously, without warning, as in sudden death.

INTERVENTION
1. Initiate CPR.
2. Immediately defibrillate at 200 joules (delivered energy) and proceed with standing orders.

ADDITIONAL EXAMPLES

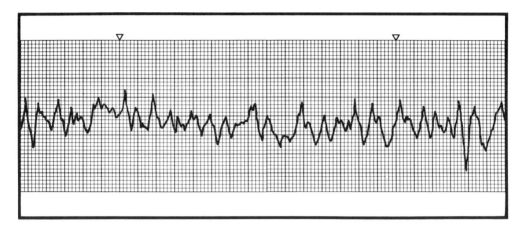

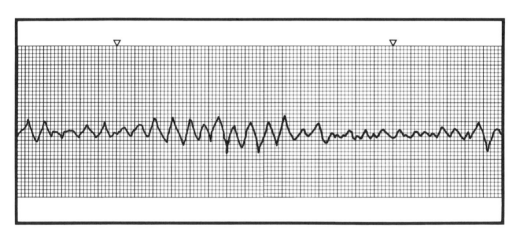

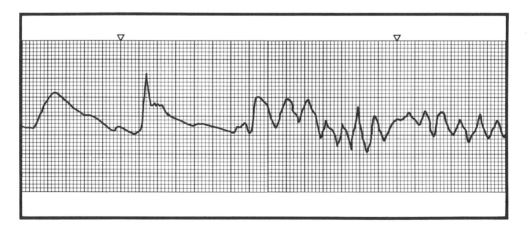

Idioventricular Rhythm

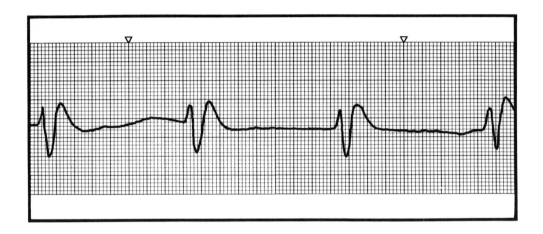

CHARACTERISTICS
1. **QRS Complexes:**
   a. Wide and varied.
   b. Conduction greater than 0.12 seconds.
   c. Uniform shape.
   d. Irregular rhythm.
2. **P Waves:** Absent.
3. **Rate:** Ventricular rate 40 per minute.

SIGNIFICANCE
This rhythm occurs when the conduction system above the ventricles fails to generate an electrical impulse. The ventricles will respond automatically, initiating an impulse to prevent asystole.

The ventricular muscle has an inherent automaticity of 30–40 beats per minute. This rate is too slow to maintain an adequate blood pressure; the patient is unconscious, often without a palable pulse.

The presence of an idioventricular rhythm may reflect severe heart disease or myocardial damage as the result of ischemia or muscle death. This rhythm is commonly seen immediately after defibrillation.

INTERVENTION
1. Determine level of consciousness.
2. Assess adequate airway and ventilation.
3. Verify presence or absence of pulse and provide basic life support as indicated.

4. If the heart rate is less than 60 and the patient is unconscious, initiate and continue CPR until more appropriate, definitive care is available.
5. Periodically stop CPR to assess rhythm.
6. If rate increases, check for pulse and blood pressure. Continue CPR if pulse remains less than 60 and patient remains unconscious.

ADDITIONAL EXAMPLES

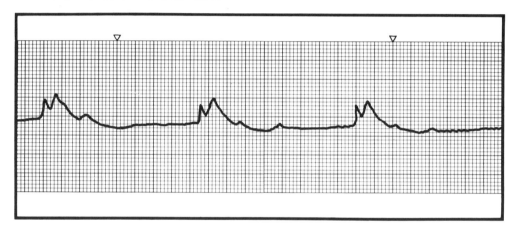

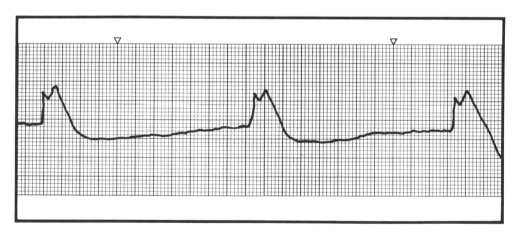

Asystole

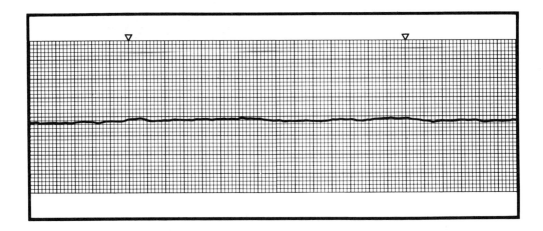

CHARACTERISTICS
The absence of any complexes indicates complete cessation of electrical activity. The heart lies motionless and the ECG will record a straight line pattern.

SIGNIFICANCE
Unlike ventricular fibrillation, which is often reversed with defibrillation, asystole is a very grave situation. If CPR is not initiated within the first four minutes, irreversible cellular death will occur, clouding any hope of resuscitation.

INTERVENTION
1. Initiate CPR immediately.
2. Verify rhythm as asystole and not ventricular fibrillation.
   a. Check calibration.
   b. Check leads and cable.
3. Continue CPR until paramedics arrive or during patient transport.

Pacemakers (Paced Rhythm)

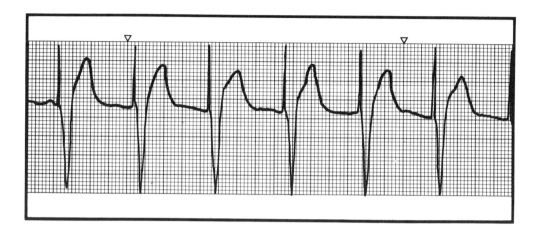

CHARACTERISTICS

A pacemaker is a battery-operated device used to artificially induce an electrical impulse in the ailing heart. The most common use of pacemakers is for situations in which the heart rate is so slow that the patient experiences lightheadedness, fainting, dizziness, or hypotension. In extreme cases, a permanent pacemaker is implanted in the chest, usually below either clavicle and directly beneath the skin, making it quite visible. It is about the size of a pack of cigarettes.

The pacemaker consists of two components: a battery source and wire electrode. The electrode is attached to either the inside or outside of the right ventricle. An electrical impulse is fired through the electrode to the heart muscle, causing a wave of depolarization to spread through the ventricles, thereby causing a mechanical contraction heart beat.

Because the impulse is fired so rapidly from the pacemaker, the ECG shows only a sharp, pointed deflection, immediately followed by a QRS complex. Since the impulse originated within the ventricles but outside the normal conduction pathway, the QRS complex will be abnormally wide and bizarre looking.

SIGNIFICANCE

Several things can happen to interfere with the proper functioning of a pacemaker. A low battery will cause the pacemaker rate to slow. If the rate is too slow, the patient may become symptomatic.

Excessive scarring near the tip of the electrode, dislodged wires, or faulty equipment can cause failure of the pacemaker to effectively stimulate the ventricles. This is seen when a pacemaker spike is present but no QRS complex follows.

Loss of the QRS complex signifies that the ventricles are not being stimulated and there is no mechanical contraction or movement of blood. If this persists, cardiac arrest ensues.

INTERVENTION

1. Assess the patient for level of consciousness, presence of respirations, and pulse.
2. If cardiac arrest is determined, initiate CPR.
3. If the patient is unconscious and his/her pulse or systolic blood pressure is less than 60, begin CPR.
4. If there is evidence of pacemaker function and the patient is conscious, but complaining of lightheadedness, dizziness, or angina, support with oxygen and continue to monitor patient's vital signs while awaiting paramedics.

ADDITIONAL EXAMPLES

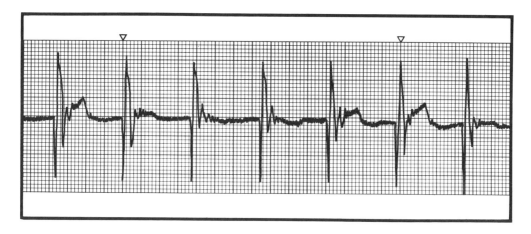

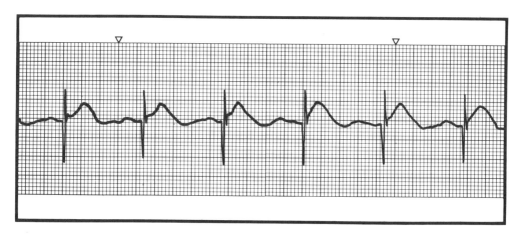

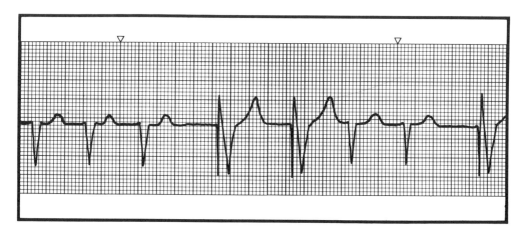

Artifact

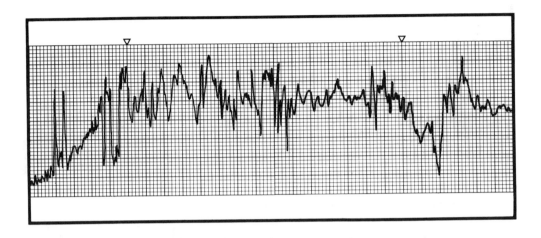

CHARACTERISTICS/SIGNIFICANCE

Artifact is any external disturbance that alters or distorts the electrical signal of the ECG display. Such disturbance can significantly interfere with accurate interpretation, as artifact can in some cases mimick arrhythmias. Common causes of ECG artifact are

1. Alternating current generators that produce 60-cycle (Hertz) interference, i.e., electric blankets, high-voltage towers, fluorescent lights.
2. Involuntary muscle tremors or seizure activity which will cause small erratic waves in the baseline.
3. Patient movement, which causes the baseline to wander up and down (often referred to as a wandering baseline).
4. Poor contact between skin and electrode, or defective cables, which cause chaotic and irregular deflections in the baseline that may be mistaken for atrial or ventricular fibrillation.

INTERVENTION

Every attempt must be made to correct or eliminate the presence of artifact before the rhythm is identified, and every precaution must be taken to ensure that what is seen as ventricular fibrillation is not artifact in disguise. Never defibrillate when artifact is present.

MUSCLE TREMOR

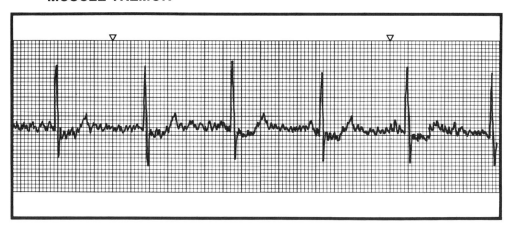

WANDERING BASELINE

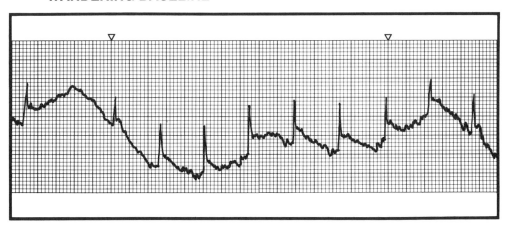

LOOSE ELECTRODE OR DEFECTIVE CABLE

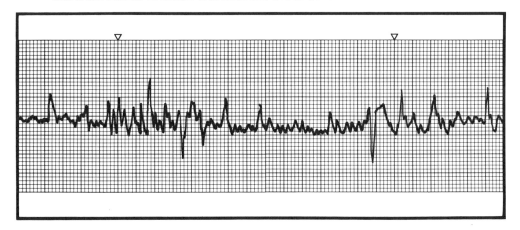

SIXTY-CYCLE INTERFERENCE

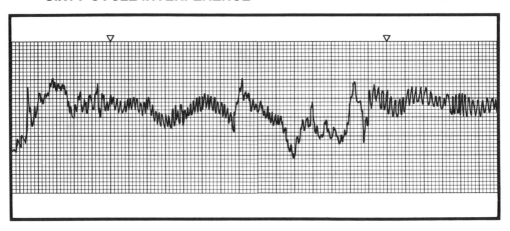

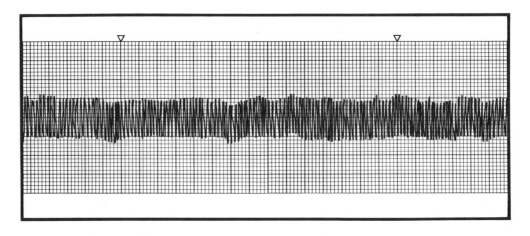

Appendix 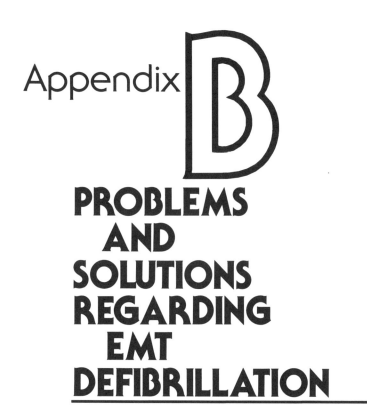 **B**

PROBLEMS AND SOLUTIONS REGARDING EMT DEFIBRILLATION

PROBLEM	CAUSE/SOLUTION
1. Flashing red light on monitoring unit.	a. Change battery pack. b. Battery memory developed secondary to improper use— less likely to develop the more it is used. Batteries in infrequent use should be routinely recycled; refer to SOP under equipment maintenance.
2. Paper recorder does not run.	a. Defective fuse. b. Battery discharged below operating level. c. Defective paper-drive motor.
3. No trace on paper.	a. Stylus heat too low. b. Defective stylus.
4. Luminous trace on cardioscope fades or is absent.	a. Battery discharged below operating level; replace battery.
5. Forgot to close tape door; event not recorded.	a. Provide explanation on incident report and submit with ECG strip.
6. Excessive 60-cycle interference.	a. Electrical appliances in vicinity, i.e., electric blankets, fluorescent lights, high-voltage wires. Unplug appliances or move to different location.
7. Excessive artifact.	a. Defective leads. b. Loose lead. c. Poor skin contact. d. Dry electrode. e. Patient movement. f. Defective cable.
8. Dry electrode due to outdated patches or improper packaging.	a. Replace leads. b. Use small amount of gel under patches.
9. Poor skin contact because of sweaty or wet patient; hairy chest; small, bony patient.	a. Clean skin surface with alcohol and dry with 4 x 4 gauze. b. Shave portion of chest. c. Reposition leads on arms or shoulder blades.

10. Stored energy is not delivered to the patient when both paddle push-buttons are depressed.

   a. Accidentally depressing power button instead of discharge buttons.

   b. Battery discharged below operating level; replace battery.

   c. Unit not fully charged to selected energy.

   d. Changing energy setting will dump load.

   e. Check charge light indicator; unit will bleed down if energy not delivered within 30 seconds.

11. Charge indicator shows no response or fails to reach desired stored energy level.

   a. Low battery; change battery.

12. Charge time exceeds 10 seconds to reach 200 joules.

   a. Low battery

13. No replacement battery—low battery on defibrillator unit.

   a. Rotate batteries: monitor→defibrillator→monitor.

14. Using loaner equipment without cassette recorder.

   a. Run paper recorder for documentation.

15. Defibrillating in the rain.

   a. Move patient to dry quarters.

   b. Dry patient off and ensure good paddle contact on patient's chest.

16. Authority of bystander physician.

   a. Ask for physician identification.

   b. Physician may assume responsibility if he or she specifically requests.

   c. Do not exceed your three shocks. The physician may deliver additional shocks.

   d. Observe additional shocks to make sure safe practices are followed.

17. Paramedics or doctor want ECG strip.

   a. The ECG strip is required to document initial rhythm and before/after each defibrillation. A portion can be sent with the paramedics, saving that portion which identifies initial rhythm and resulting rhythm following defibrillation.

18. Patient arrested after arrival of EMTs.

    a. Initiate CPR and, once stable, attach monitor and begin recording.

    b. Enact treatment according to standing orders.

19. Defibrillating during transport of patient.

    a. Vehicle must come to a complete stop and the rhythm must be reassessed. Defibrillate only when the vehicle is stopped.

Appendix 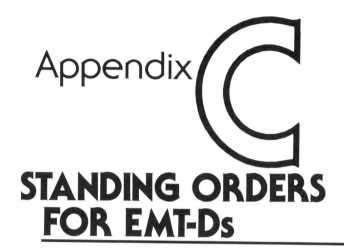 C

STANDING ORDERS FOR EMT-Ds

Purpose: The purpose of these orders is to provide prompt defibrillation for patients who have confirmed circulatory arrest due to ventricular fibrillation.

Authorization: In the event of a cardiac arrest, I authorize you to perform the following:

1. Immediately upon arrival, verify circulatory and respiratory arrest by the absence of consciousness, respiration and *carotid pulse.*

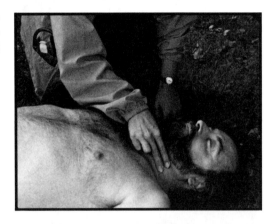

2. Initiate CPR and the Defibrillation protocol:
   a. *Two-man response team:* one EMT initiates one-person CPR using mouth-to-mask ventilations, and continues this role throughout the resuscitation. The other EMT becomes the *"Defibrillator-EMT" directing the resuscitation, and operating the defibrillator.
   b. *Three or more response team:* two EMTs initiate two-person CPR using bag-valve-mask and continue this role throughout the resuscitation. The other EMT becomes the *"Defibrillator-EMT" directing the resuscitation, and operating the defibrillator.

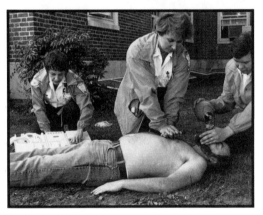

3. Turn on monitor and recorder; give a verbal report:
   a. identify yourself and responding fire department.
   b. describe the situation.
   c. report each step as you proceed through the standing orders.
   d. continue to report what is happening as it occurs, i.e., having difficulty with airway secondary to vomitus; paramedics have arrived; moving patient, etc.
4. Calibrate machine, connect patient cable to monitor.

*The "Defibrillator-EMT": upon arrival at the scene, and verification of cardiac arrest, the Defibrillator-EMT does *not* wait for CPR to be performed for any set period of time, but proceeds immediately with the defibrillation protocols outlined in these standing orders.

5. Attach the leads, while verbally identifying their position; "white to right shoulder, black or green to left shoulder, red to left lower ribs."

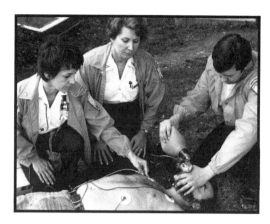

6. Remove and gel the paddles, charge to 200 joules, start the paper recorder (refer to #10), stop CPR and assess the rhythm taking no longer than 10 seconds:

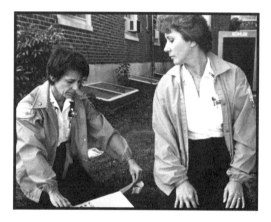

A. *THE INITIAL RHYTHM IS VENTRICULAR FIBRILLATION:* place the gelled paddles on the chest, yell "clear" and deliver a countershock. DO NOT immediately resume CPR, but assess the postshock rhythm, taking no longer than 15 seconds:*

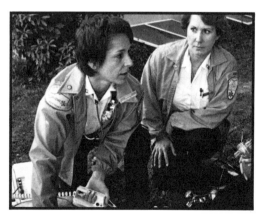

---

*If a delay of 15 seconds or more is encountered due to battery problems, artifact, uncertainty of rhythm, etc., resume CPR until the problem is resolved and then reassess.

(1) *The postshock rhythm is ventricular fibrillation:* Immediately charge the paddles, clear and shock a second time. Resume CPR for up to 30 seconds; recharge the paddles; then reassess the rhythm.

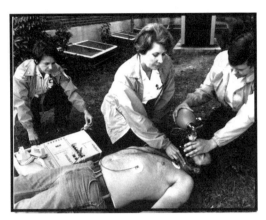

    (a) *Still ventricular fibrillation:* clear and shock a third and final time. Resume CPR for up to 30 seconds. Check the rhythm. If ventricular fibrillation continues after the third shock, continue CPR until the paramedics arrive, or the patient is transported to an emergency facility.

    (b) *Asystole or non-perfusing*:* Resume CPR for up to 30 seconds and then reassess.

    (c) *Perfusing rhythm with palpable carotid pulse:* check for respirations and blood pressure. If present, continue to monitor and administer oxygen.

(2) *The postshock rhythm is asystole or non-perfusing*:* Resume CPR for up to 30 seconds and then reassess. If rhythm returns to ventricular fibrillation proceed with step 6-(1a).

(3) *The postshock rhythm produces a palpable carotid pulse:* check for respirations and blood pressure. If present, continue to monitor and administer oxygen.

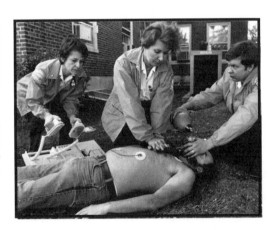

---

*A non-perfusing rhythm exists when complexes are seen, but a carotid pulse is absent.

B. *THE INITIAL RHYTHM IS ASYS-TOLE:* Resume CPR for up to 30 seconds while you:
   (1) Check leads and patient cable connections.
   (2) Check calibrations.
   Then stop CPR and reassess:
      (a) *The rhythm is now ventricular fibrillation:* go to ventricular fibrillation sequence above in 6.a.
      (b) *The rhythm is still asystole or non-perfusing*:* resume 2-man CPR and reassess periodically.

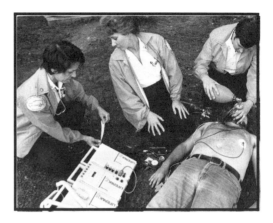

C. *THE INITIAL RHYTHM IS NEITHER VENTRICULAR FIBRILLATION NOR ASYSTOLE* and circulatory arrest persists: continue CPR for up to 30 seconds and then reassess rhythm and pulse.
   (1) *The rhythm becomes ventricular fibrillation:* go to the ventricular fibrillation sequence above in 6.a.
   (2) *A rhythm and pulse have returned:* check for respirations and blood pressure and continue to monitor.
   (3) *A pulse is absent but rhythm is not ventricular fibrillation:* resume 2-man CPR until paramedics arrive and reassess periodically.

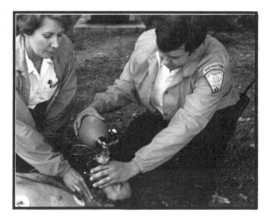

7. *No more than a total of three (3) countershocks will be given during a resuscitation by EMTs, except for the following single exception:*
   a. If the third countershock above produced a *perfusing* rhythm, AND after a period of time, the patient goes back into ventricular fibrillation, *one* more countershock may be delivered according to the procedure described above.
8. CPR should not cease for more than 15 seconds when assessing the rhythm.

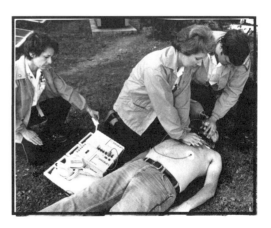

---

*A non-perfusing rhythm exists when complexes are seen, but a carotid pulse is absent.

9. If the patient's systolic blood pressure is less than 60, and the patient remains unconscious, continue CPR.

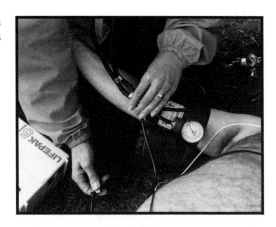

10. The paper strip should be obtained each time the rhythm is assessed, before and after each countershock is given, and whenever there is a return of any electrical activity. In other words, a paper recording should be obtained whenever CPR is stopped to determine the rhythm. Mail the rhythm strip, tape recording and incident form to the E.M.S. Office within 24 hours.

11. Reassess the rhythm following the second, third and/or fourth countershock within 30 seconds.

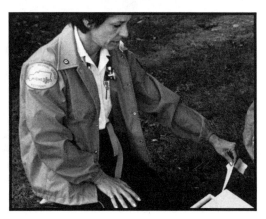

12. Always check for a carotid pulse before taking the blood pressure. If you cannot palpate a carotid pulse, initiate CPR immediately.

13. Frequent monitoring of the rhythm is necessary anytime a perfusing rhythm is restored with defibrillation since the patient is at high risk to lapse back into ventricular fibrillation. Monitor vital signs at frequent intervals of 3-5 minutes and record on the flow sheet.

14. Continue the administration of oxygen and support ventilations as indicated in patients who have been resuscitated.

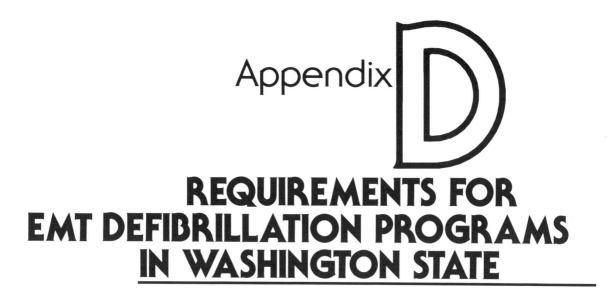

Appendix D

REQUIREMENTS FOR
EMT DEFIBRILLATION PROGRAMS
IN WASHINGTON STATE

I. The Physician Director's Role
   A. The Medical Director must be a physician licensed to practice in the state of Washington.
   B. The Medical Director is responsible for close medical supervision of the program and maintaining high skill level and performance of EMTs trained to defibrillate, including:
      1. Permission for EMTs to participate in the program;
      2. Written authorization of standing orders;
      3. Supervision of continuing education and quarterly evaluations;
      4. Review and documentation of each case using electronic voice and ECG recordings of treatments performed in the field;
      5. Establishment and maintenance of individual case records;
      6. Removal of permission for EMTs to participate for any of the following reasons:
         a. Nonprofessional behavior or attitude;
         b. Nonadherence to standing orders;
         c. Nonattendance of mandatory continuing education classes;
         d. Failure to demonstrate high performance or skill levels.

II. Selection of Candidates for Training
   A. All candidates must be EMTs with current certification.
   B. All candidates must be recommended for training by their employer or designated supervisor.
   C. All candidates must be able to perform perfect CPR as judged by the Medical Director or his designee.

III. Training Requirements
   See the enclosed Instructor's Course Outline and Student Syllabus for details of training.

IV. Continuing Education
   A. To continue to participate in the program, EMTs must attend four 2–3 hour continuing education classes per year.
   B. Continuing education classes should include:
      1. The theory and technique of defibrillation;
      2. Equipment drills;
      3. Knowledge of standing orders;
      4. Written and practical examinations, including CPR.

V. Equipment
   Defibrillators used in EMT Defibrillation Programs must be capable of making continuous voice and ECG recordings in the field for later case-review purposes.

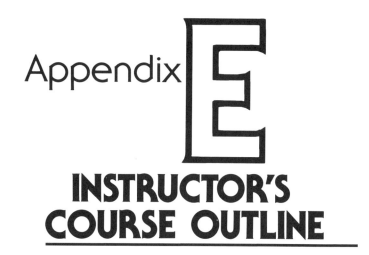

Appendix **E**

INSTRUCTOR'S
COURSE OUTLINE

This material is utilized in most EMT Defibrillation courses in Washington State.

I. Introduction

As piloted in King County, Washington, in 1978, the training of EMTs to recognize ventricular fibrillation and treat with defibrillatory shock can be completed in about 10 hours of classroom and laboratory work. This training time may be conveniently broken into three separate class periods which include: CPR Review (three hours), Didactic Lecture (three hours), and Defibrillation Laboratory (four hours). The dog defibrillation section of the laboratory is optional. Since the necessary facilities may not be immediately available to all training programs, it may be necessary to arrange this laboratory experience at another location. Teaching assistants should be ACLS personnel such as paramedics or CCU nurses.

II. CPR Review Session (three hours)
   A. Description

   Cardiopulmonary resuscitation is the fundamental life-sustaining treatment provided by the EMT for cases of cardiac arrest. CPR provides the foundation upon which any potential improvements in EMT care rest. For this reason, the ability of all trainees to peform CPR to strict American Heart Association standards should be prerequisite to any further training.

   The CPR Review Session utilizes recording manikins and requires all trainees to demonstrate optimal one- and two-person CPR technique. One manikin should be reserved for remedial instruction since most trainees who don't meet the standards initially can be trained up to standard with individual tutoring by the end of the session.
   B. Materials and Personnel
      1. One instructor/six trainees
      2. One and a half recording manikins/six trainees
   C. Instructor's Tasks
      1. Prepare general course introduction and schedule.
      2. Prepare student syllabus packets for distribution.
      3. Assure that equipment and supplies are available and in working condition.
      4. Brief teaching assistants regarding their roles and responsibilities during the session.
      5. Before completing the session, make sure that all trainees can perform the skills to standards.

III. Didactic Lecture Session (three hours)
   A. Description
      A complete outline of lecture topics appears in the attached Student Syllabus section. Presentation may be enhanced by selecting appropriate slides from the American Heart Association collection or by using other teaching aids. The defibrillator may be illustrated with slides as well as by actual demonstration. The defibrillator operation section should be revised to describe the defibrillator utilized by your program.
   B. Materials and Personnel
      1. Lecturer (Medical Director)
      2. One teaching assistant/30 trainees
      3. One defibrillator
      4. Optional slide projector and cardiac slides
   C. Instructor's Tasks
      1. Review the lesson outline.
      2. Use references and your own experience to enrich the lesson outlines when you deliver your lecture.
      3. Select or prepare appropriate instructional aids (i.e., AHA slides).
      4. Assure that equipment and supplies are available and in working condition.

IV. Defibrillation Laboratory (four hours)
   A. Description
      The defibrillation laboratory provides "hands-on" training and practice with the defibrillator. The laboratory may be organized around training stations, each of which emphasizes different aspects of the training. Each station is staffed by a teaching assistant who works with about 10 trainees at a time. Teaching assistants should simulate problems that might occur in the field. If the dog lab option is chosen, it becomes one of the stations. Groups of 10 trainees then rotate between the following stations:
      1. At the *Defibrillator Components and Operation* station, trainees learn
         a. How to operate the defibrillator
         b. How to calibrate the machine
         c. Defibrillator maintenance
         d. Defibrillator safety
         e. Defibrillator supplies
      2. At the *Rhythm Recognition* station, trainees learn to monitor the ECG in conjunction with ongoing CPR and to recognize artifact and ventricular fibrillation on an arrhythmia manikin.

3. At the *Standing Orders Review* station, trainees practice on an arrhythmia manikin:
   a. Continuity of patient assessment
   b. Continuity of basic life support
   c. Short time intervals for patient assessment and resumption of CPR
   d. Talking into the tape recorder
   e. Administering no more than three countershocks.
4. Optional *Dog Defibrillation* station
   If facilities for animal care and anesthesia are available, this station can provide the trainee with the experience of delivering DC shock to a living creature. This experience can boost trainee confidence and better prepare them for actual delivery of care in the field.
   This section should be staffed by a technician, veterinarian, or physician responsible for animal care and anesthesia. Ventricular fibrillation is induced in the anesthetized dogs by means of an electronic device obtained from the defibrillator manufacturer. Each trainee should deliver at least one shock in attempting to defibrillate the animal.
B. Materials and Personnel
   1. Each training station should include
      One instructor/10 trainees
      One arrhythmia manikin/10 trainees
      One defibrillator/10 trainees
      (NOTE: *Actual shock should be administered to manikins at no more than 40 joules or they may be damaged.*)
   2. The dog defibrillation station should include
      One animal care and anesthesia technician
      One instructor/10 trainees
      One anesthetized dog/10 trainees
      One ventricular fibrillation inducer
      One defibrillator
C. Instructor's Tasks
   1. Prepare brief review of lecture topics.
   2. Assure that necessary equipment and supplies are available and in working order.
   3. Brief all teaching assistants regarding their roles and responsibilities during the laboratory.
   4. Before completing the lab, make sure that all students can perform the skills.

V. Testing
   The final exam night should be scheduled following the defibrillation laboratory. The written exam can be administered to one group of trainees while another group completes the

practical exam. Practical testing should be supervised by the medical director and can be accomplished using an arrhythmia manikin. Each trainee should be required to set up the monitor, recognize ventricular fibrillation, and administer defibrillatory shock safely and appropriately while one- or two-person CPR is underway.

VI. Medical Supervision
Defibrillation is a medical procedure that presents serious potential danger to the patient and to the EMT. Medical authority and accountability are required to begin or continue an EMT Defibrillation Program. Physician directorship of such a program is mandatory. The program Medical Director should take responsibility for EMT defibrillation training, ongoing monitoring of cases treated by EMT-D (tapes), evaluation of EMT-D personnel, continuing education for EMT-Ds, and signing of EMT-D standing orders. An EMT defibrillation program should also have a professional coordinator to act as liaison person between the various administrative units involved and to handle the day-to-day management of the program.

VII. Continuing Education
Degradation of rarely performed skills is a problem for responders at all levels. Continuing education, equipment drills, and supervision are necessary to maintain an EMT/Defibrillation program. Quarterly ongoing education sessions, with evaluation, are recommended to assess skill levels and attitudes of each EMT/D.

VIII. Removal of Permission
The medical director has the responsibility of authorizing participation and also may revoke this authority for the following:
A. Nonprofessional behavior or attitude.
B. Nonadherence to standing orders.
C. Nonattendance of mandatory continuing education classes.
D. Failure to demonstrate high performance skill level training.

Appendix F

PRACTICE RHYTHMS

1.

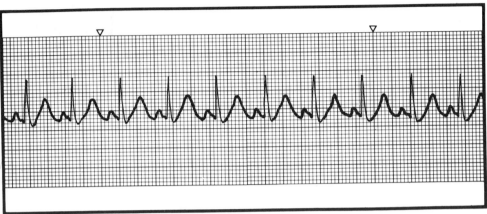

2.

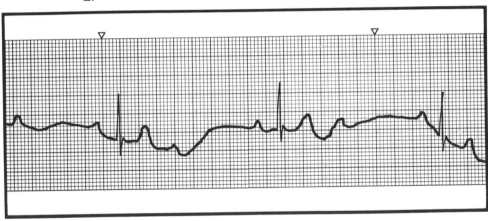

3.

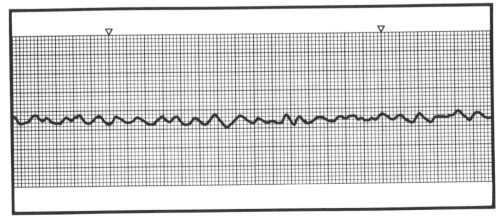

4.

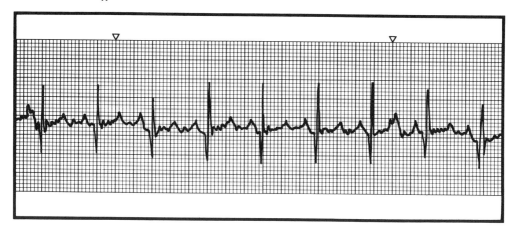

5.

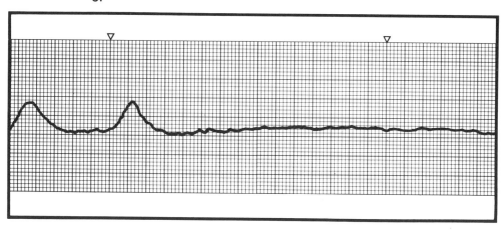

6.

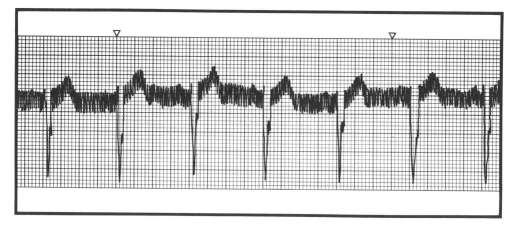

7.

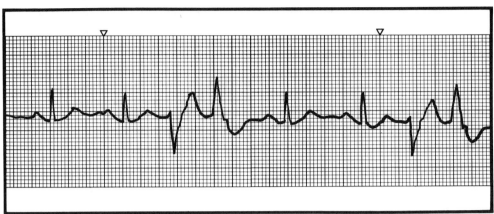

8.

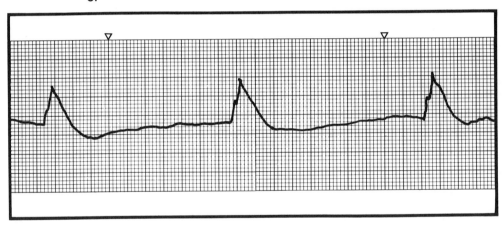

9.

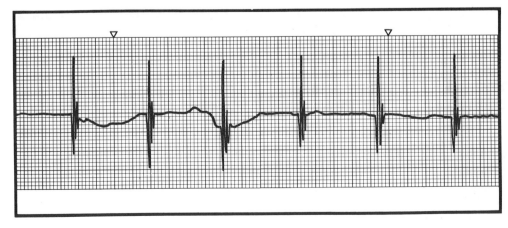

10.

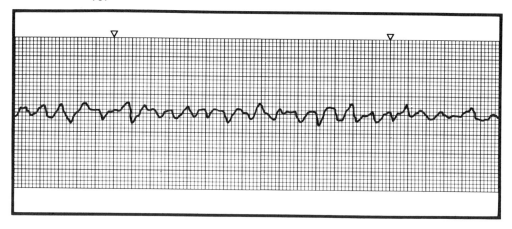

11.

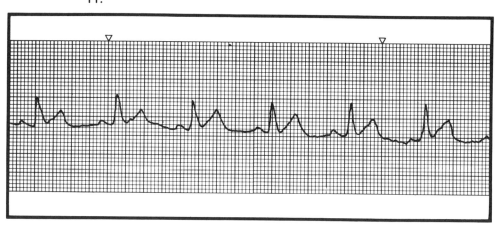

12.

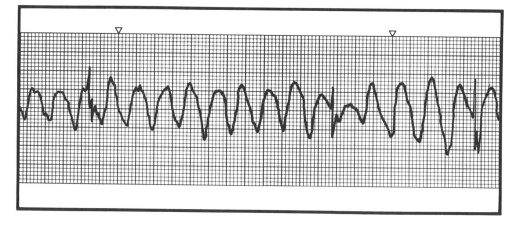

13.

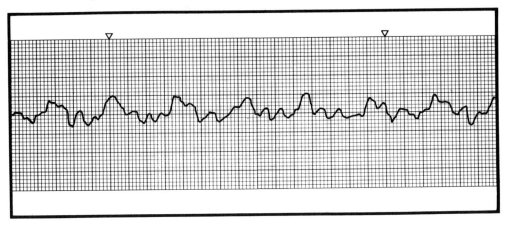

14.

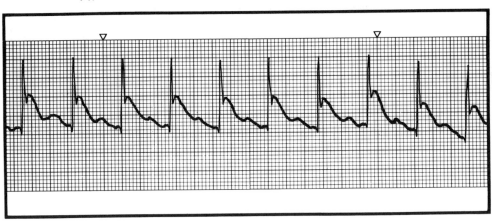

15.

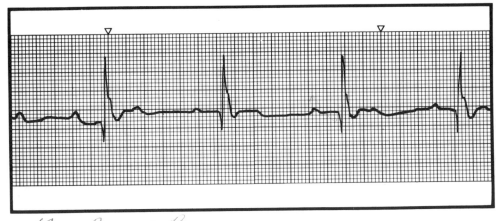

1° = P ———→ R
2°-1 = dropped QRS
2°-2 = q2 q3 dropped QRS
3° =

16.

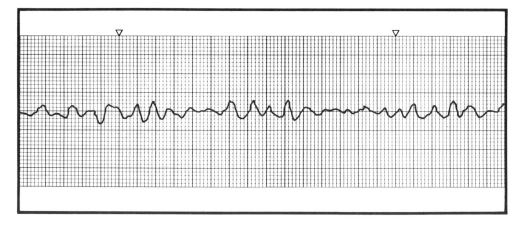

17.

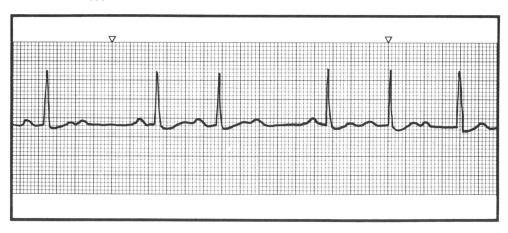

18.

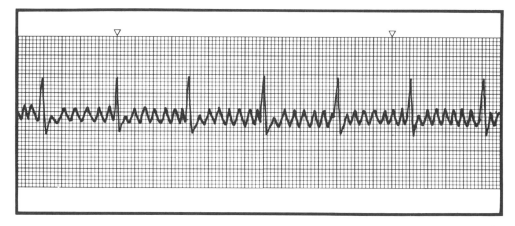

19.

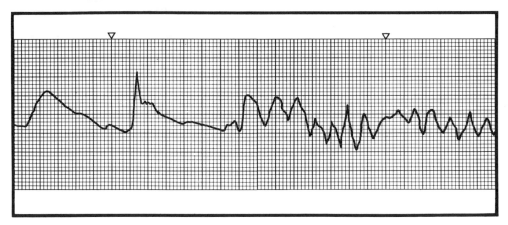

20.

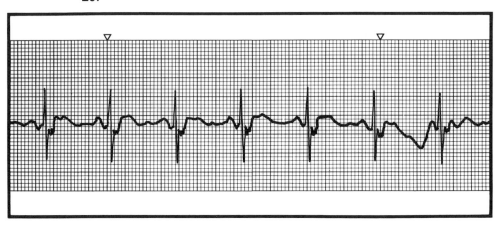

21.

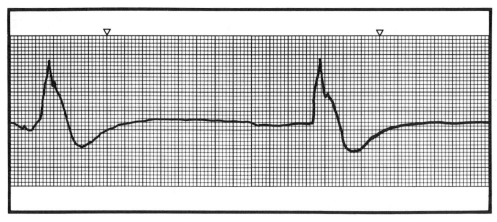

22.

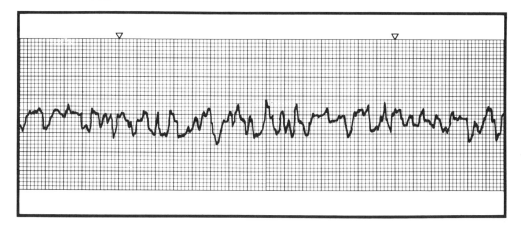

23.

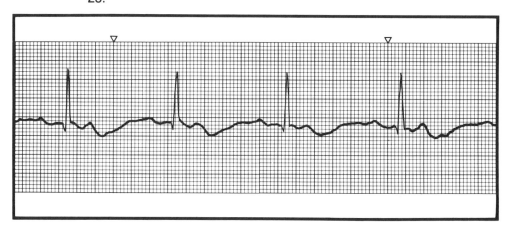

24.

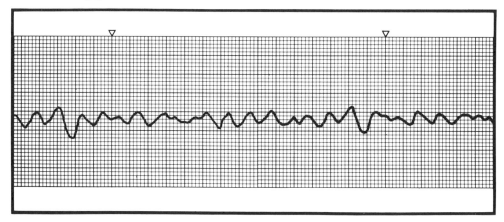

25.

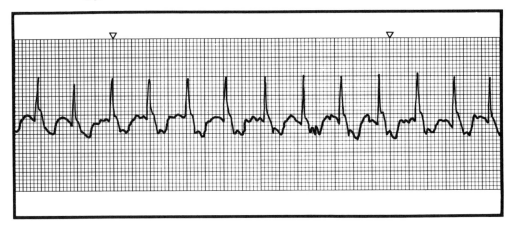

26.

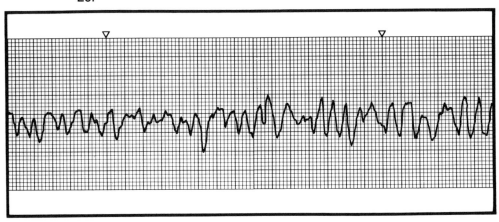

27.

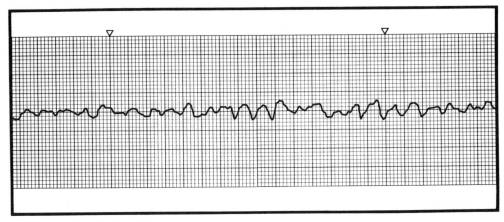

28.

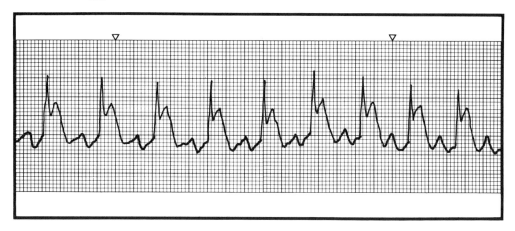

29.

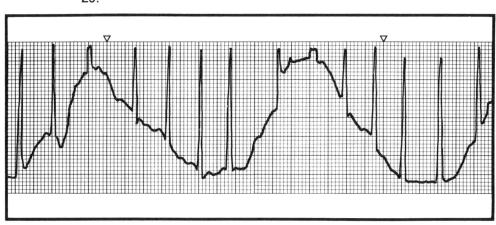

30.

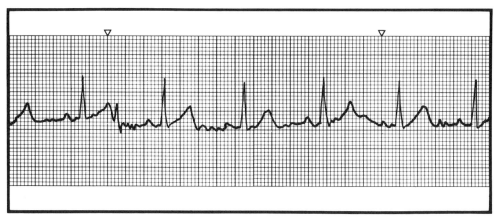

31.

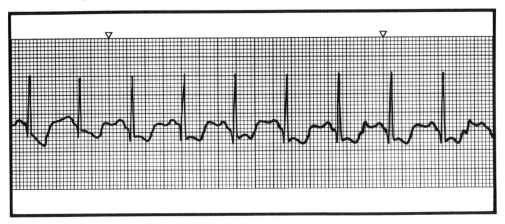

32.

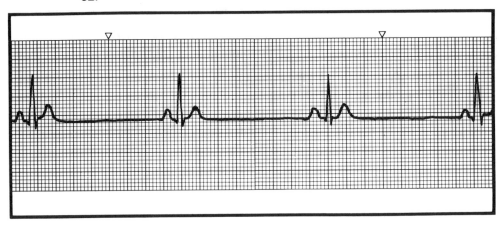

33.

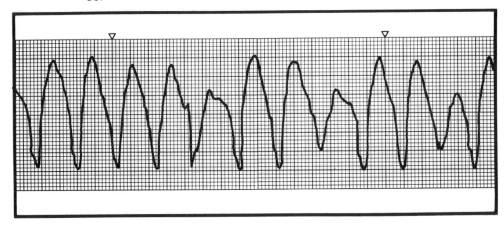

34.

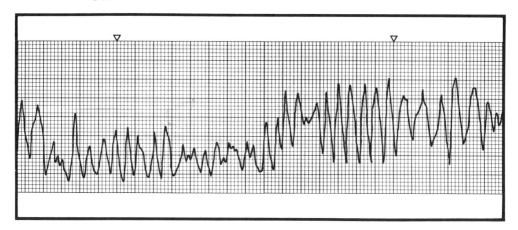

35.

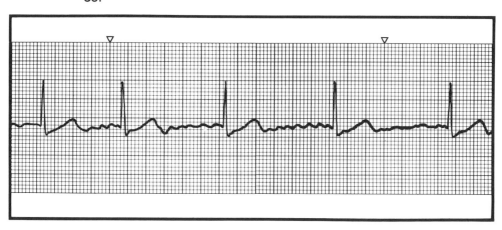

36.

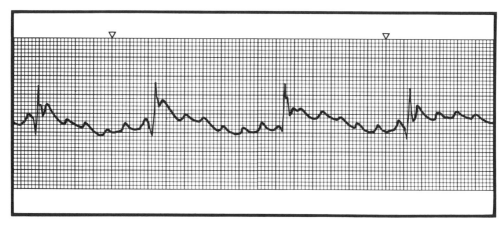

37.

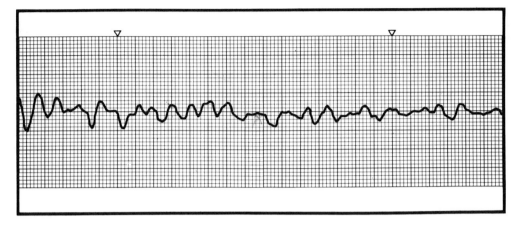

38.

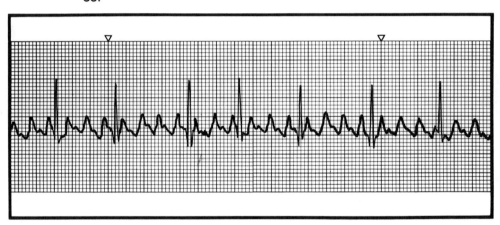

39.

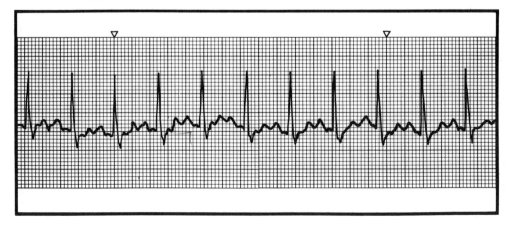

40.

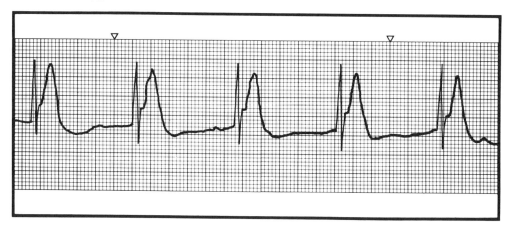

41.

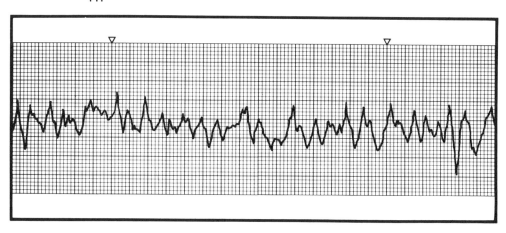

42.

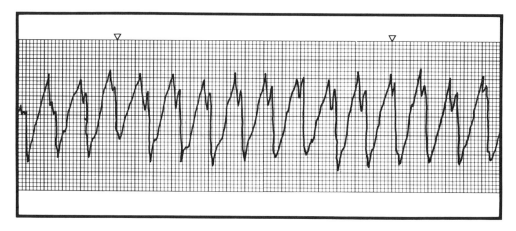

43.

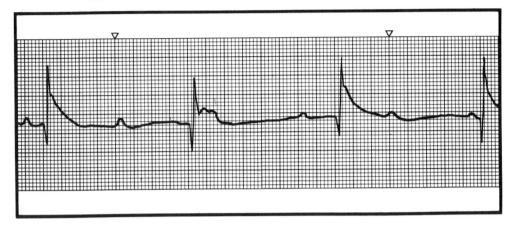

44.

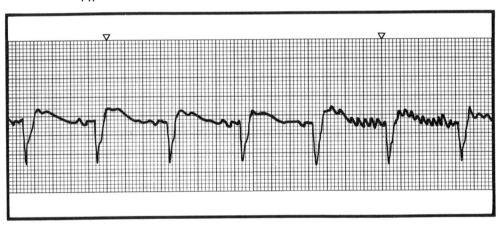

45.

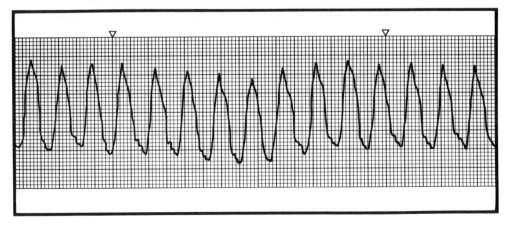

46.

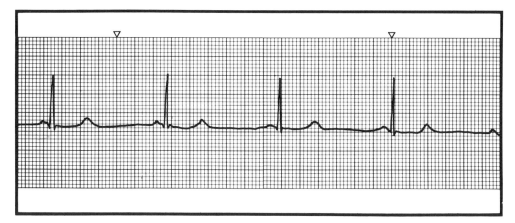

47.

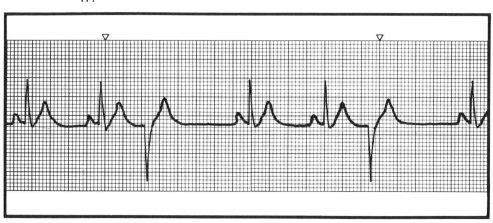

48.

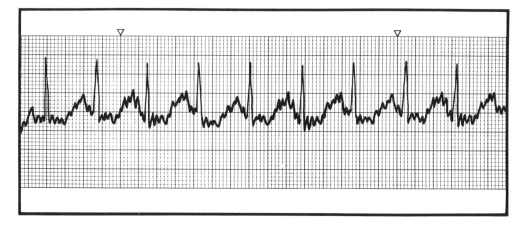

49.

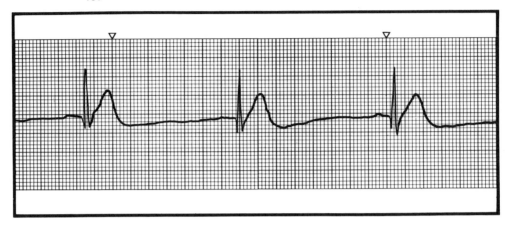

50.

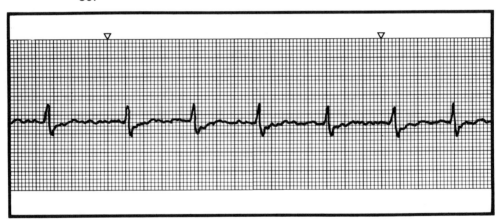

51.

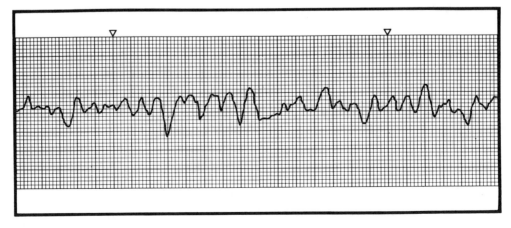

Practice Rhythms: Answers

1. Sinus tachycardia
2. Second-degree heart block, Mobitz type II
3. Fine ventricular fibrillation
4. Normal sinus rhythm with artifact
5. Asystole
6. Artifact: 60-cycle interference
7. Normal sinus rhythm with coupled PVC
8. Idioventricular rhythm
9. Pacemaker spikes without conduction
10. Ventricular fibrillation
11. Normal sinus rhythm
12. Ventricular flutter
13. Ventricular fibrillation
14. First-degree heart block
15. Second-degree heart block, Mobitz type II
16. Ventricular fibrillation
17. Second-degree heart block, Wenckebach
18. Atrial flutter
19. Ventricular fibrillation
20. Normal sinus rhythm
21. Idioventricular rhythm
22. Ventricular fibrillation
23. First-degree heart block
24. Ventricular fibrillation
25. Supraventricular tachycardia
26. Ventricular fibrillation
27. Ventricular fibrillation
28. First-degree heart block
29. Supraventricular tachycardia with wandering baseline
30. Normal sinus rhythm
31. Sinus tachycardia
32. Sinus bradycardia
33. Ventricular tachycardia
34. Coarse ventricular fibrillation
35. Atrial fibrillation
36. Atrial flutter
37. Ventricular fibrillation
38. Atrial flutter
39. Sinus tachycardia
40. Nodal rhythm
41. Ventricular fibrillation

42. Ventricular tachycardia
43. Third-degree heart block
44. Normal sinus rhythm with artifact
45. Ventricular tachycardia
46. Sinus bradycardia
47. Normal sinus rhythm with premature ventricular contractions
48. Sinus tachycardia with artifact and wandering baseline
49. Sinus bradycardia
50. Atrial fibrillation
51. Ventricular fibrillation

GLOSSARY

Glossary

acidosis An excess of acid in the blood.

alternating current Electrical current that reverses direction at regular intervals.

amplitude The size or strength of the electrical deflection on the ECG recording.

angina Acute pain in the chest caused by a temporary interruption in the blood supply to the heart muscle.

apex The anatomical portion of the heart that lies directly above the diaphragm.

arrhythmia Any rhythm other than a normal sinus rhythm.

arteriosclerosis A disease of the blood vessels, which become thickened and narrowed, reducing blood flow to body tissues.

artifact Extraneous mechanical or electrical interference to the ECG signal.

asynchronization A lack of organized sequence.

asystole A flat ECG in which there is no electrical activity.

atrial fibrillation An abnormal rhythm in which the atria are firing chaotically without contraction. The ventricles continue to beat in a coordinated fashion, maintaining BP and pulse.

atrial flutter An abnormal rhythm in the atrium, repetitively and rapidly depolarized from an ectopic focus originating in the atria. The rhythm generally resembles a sawtooth pattern.

atrioventricular node (AV node) That portion of the conduction system located between the atria and ventricles which receives an impulse from the SA node and then transmits that impulse to the bundle of His.

atrium (pl: atria) One of two superior chambers of the heart resting atop the ventricles. The atria receive the blood from the body and lungs and then channel the blood to the ventricles.

automaticity The ability of any portion of the conduction system or heart muscle to initiate an electrical impulse.

baseline	That portion of the electrocardiogram that is iso-electric, or without electrical activity.
bradycardia	An arrhythmia in which the heart rate is less than 60 beats per minute.
bundle branches	That portion of the conduction system which divides below the bundle of His into right and left branches.
bundle of His	That portion of the electrical conduction system which receives the impulse from the AV node, passing it along to the bundle branches.
calibration	The adjustment of amplitude of the electric signal on the monitor. Sometimes called *gain.*
capacitor	Part of the defibrillator in which the electrical current is generated and stored until delivered to the patient.
coarse ventricular fibrillation	Ventricular fibrillation in which the fibrillatory waves are stronger than in fine ventricular fibrillation.
complete heart block	The most serious type of heart block, this represents a complete interruption in the transmission of an impulse. The atria and ventricles are contracting independently of one another. Also called *third-degree heart block.*
conductivity	Transmission of an electrical impulse by way of specialized tissue.
configuration	The shape of the various ECG waves.
coronary arteries	Those that supply the heart muscle with oxygenated blood. A blockage or narrowing of the coronary arteries will result in a loss of blood flow to the heart muscle and death to the tissue.
couplets	The occurrence of two premature ventricular contractions side-by-side. Also called *coupling.*
defibrillation	The delivery of an electric current through the chest wall and heart for the purpose of terminating ventricular fibrillation.
defibrillator	The device used for defibrillation.

deflection	A deviation from the isoelectric baseline, such as a wave or complex.
depolarization	An electrical process in which the spread of an impulse through the myocardium changes the electrical charges on the surface of the muscle, causing a mechanical contraction to occur.
direct current	An electrical current that flows in one direction.
ectopic beat	One that originates outside the normal conduction pathway.
ectopic focus	The site of an ectopic beat.
electrical death	Occurs when normal heart rhythm changes to a fatal rhythm and the heart stops pumping blood, resulting in sudden cardiac arrest.
electrical lead	*See* lead.
electrocardiogram (ECG or EKG)	A graphic recording of the heart's electrical activity.
electrodes	Electrical devices or patches placed on the exterior surface of the body. Electrical leads coming from the electrocardiograph are connected to the electrodes, allowing the reception and transmission of electrical impulses to the electrocardiogram.
electrophysiology	The study of the electrical forces of the heart.
fine ventricular fibrillation	Ventricular fibrillation in which the amplitude of the fibrillatory waves is dampened.
first-degree heart block	A delayed impulse conduction from the SA node to the AV node, represented by a PR interval > 0.20 seconds.
joule	A unit for measuring energy, used interchangeably with watt second.
lead	An arrangement of electrodes through which electrical activity from the heart is transmitted to a recording device.
mechanical contraction	One that occurs after the spread of an electrical impulse through the muscle; the heart contracts, pumping blood forward. Evidence of contraction is noted by the presence of a pulse.

millivolt	One-thousandth of a volt of electricity.
Mobitz type I	A type of second-degree heart block in which the PR interval increasingly lengthens until a beat is dropped. *Also called* Wenckebach.
Mobitz type II	A type of second-degree heart block in which a heartbeat is periodically dropped.
monitoring	1. The continuous visualization and display on a screen of the patient's cardiac rhythm. 2. Rhythm interpretation.
multifocal PVCs	Two or more premature ventricular contractions that differ in configuration.
myocardial infarction	The death of a portion of heart muscle as a result of an interruption of blood supply.
PR interval	Part of the ECG measured from the beginning of the P wave to the beginning of the QRS complex; represents the time from atrial depolarization to the beginning of ventricular depolarization.
premature ventricular contraction	An ectopic beat originating somewhere in the ventricle wall which causes an early and abnormal contraction of the heart muscle.
Purkinje fibers	Fibers located directly in the ventricular musculature, which cause the ventricles to contract.
QRS complex	Part of the ECG that represents depolarization of the ventricles; should not exceed 0.12 seconds.
repolarization	The second electrical process associated with mechanical contraction, in which the heart muscle returns to a resting state.
rhythm	The electrical activity displayed by the heart; seen as the electrocardiogram.
risk factors	Those conditions that make individuals susceptible to developing specific diseases.
septum	The heart structure that separates and divides the atria and ventricles, making each a separate chamber.
secondary pacemaker	System whereby, should the SA node fail to fire, a different focus in the atria, AV node, or ventricles can initiate a rhythm.

standard lead	The standard arrangement of electrodes: the positive lead is positioned near the left hip and the negative lead is positioned near the right shoulder. Also called *Lead II*.
sternum	The breastbone, located midline on the chest.
sudden cardiac arrest	Occurs when the heart suddenly stops pumping blood, resulting in loss of consciousness and then death unless rapid emergency care is provided.
supraventricular tachycardia	Rapid arrhythmia originating above the ventricles.
synchronized cardioversion	A function of the defibrillator whereby, utilizing a sensing mechanism, the defibrillator delivers a charge only after recognizing or sensing the QRS deflection. This mode of countershock is used only with tachycardia.
tachycardia	Any rhythm in which the heart rate is greater than 100 beats per minute.
third-degree heart block	*See* complete heart block.
T wave	Part of the ECG that follows the QRS complex and represents repolarization of the ventricles.
U wave	Part of an ECG that represents a delayed repolarization of the ventricles and, rarely seen, follows the T wave.
ventricles	The two inferior chambers of the heart, which receive blood from the atria and then pump blood to the lungs and body.
ventricular flutter	A transitional arrhythmia that occurs when ventricular tachycardia degenerates into ventricular fibrillation.
ventricular fiibrillation	A fateful arrhythmia in which there is a loss of coordinated contractions, resulting in sudden death.
ventricular tachycardia	The occurrence of three or more PVCs in a row.

watt seconds   Outdated term used for measuring energy.

waves   The positive and negative deflections of an ECG, denoting the depolarization and repolarization processes of the heart's electrical system. They include the P wave, the QRS complex, the T wave, and the U wave.

Wenckebach   See Mobitz type I.

Index